Skinny Chicks Don't Eat Salads

STOP STARVING,
START EATING. . .
STILL GET SKINNY!

CHRISTINE AVANTI

This edition first published 2009 by Rodale
an imprint of Pan Macmillan Ltd
Pan Macmillan, 20 New Wharf Road, London N1 9RR
Basingstoke and Oxford
Associated companies throughout the world
www.panmacmillan.com

ISBN 978-1-9057-44-44-2

1 3 5 7 9 8 6 4 2

A CIP catalogue record for this book is available from the British Library.

Printed and bound in the UK by CPI Mackays, Chatham ME5 8TD

This book is intended as a reference volume only, not as a medical manual. The information given here is designed to help you make informed decisions about your health. It is
not intended as a substitute for any treatment that you may have been prescribed by
your doctor. If you suspect you have a medical problem, we urge you to seek competent
medical help.

The information in this book is designed to supplement, not replace, proper exercise
training. All forms of exercise pose some inherent risks. The editors and publisher advise
readers to take full responsibility for their safety and know their limits. Before practising
the exercises in this book, be sure that your equipment is well-maintained and do not
take risks beyond your level of experience, aptitude, training and fitness. The exercise
and dietary programmes in this book are not intended as a substitute for any exercise
routine or dietary regime that may have been prescribed by your doctor. As with all
exercise and dietary programmes, you should get your doctor's approval before
beginning.

Mention of specific companies, organizations or authorities in this book does not imply
endorsement by the author or publisher, nor does mention of specific companies, organizations or authorities in the book imply that they endorse the book, its author or the
publisher.

Internet addresses given in this book were accurate at the time of going to press.

Visit **www.panmacmillan.com** to read more about all our books and to buy them. You
will also find features, author interviews and news of any author events, and you can
sign up for e-newsletters so that you're always first to hear about our new releases.

We inspire and enable people to improve their lives and the world around them

To all women who have
struggled needlessly to lose weight.
May you find peace and revelation
as you go on this journey, just like I did.

Contents

FOREWORD vi

INTRODUCTION vii

PART I: SKINNY CHICKS LEARN THE SCIENCE

1: How Salads Got Us into Big Fat Trouble 3

2: The ABCs of Weight Loss 14

3: It's the Amount That Counts 24

4: The Beauty of Balance 37

5: Munch around the Clock 46

6: Every Body's Got Issues 54

PART II: SKINNY CHICKS REVISIT PROTEIN AND CARBS

7: Lean, Mean Protein 65

8: The Carb Conspiracy 81

9: The Fat Fear Factor 91

10: Drink Yourself Skinny 105

PART III: SKINNY CHICKS PUT IT ALL TOGETHER

11: Skinny Chicks Meal Plans 117

12: Supplemental Insurance 166

13: Darnit, Get Your Lazy Butt on the Treadmill 175

PART IV: SKINNY CHICKS IN THE REAL WORLD

14: Skinny Chicks Have Their Ups and Downs 205

15: Every Day Is a Splurge Day 210

16: The Diner's Dilemma 218

17: Skinny Chicks Helpful Tricks 225

PART V: SKINNY CHICKS GET IN THE KITCHEN

RECIPES 235

APPENDIX: FOOD LISTS 275

REFERENCES 279

ACKNOWLEDGMENTS 282

INDEX 284

Foreword

A few years ago, Christine came into my office and dropped off some written information about her programme. My receptionist told me she was so nice and her materials so good that I ought to give her a call. I did, and I was so impressed with her presentation and her programme, I decided to try it myself. The more I learned about her programme, the more I realized it was not some crazy fad diet; it made sense to me as a dieter and as a physician.

One of the things I like best about this book is the way Christine explains insulin and sugar balance in a way that is physiologically correct yet easy to understand. It's a complicated subject that's not always well taught, even at medical school. But Christine puts it in such an easy-to-read format, readers will actually get it. And once you grasp the concept of insulin and blood sugar and how it relates to eating, the rest is easy. It helps you understand why you need to eat every 4 hours, why it's counterproductive to starve yourself, and how to balance your meals with the proper portions of protein, carbohydrates and fats.

Anybody can take the information in this book and apply it to his or her own life. At first, I thought it might be difficult for me. As a facial plastic and cosmetic surgeon, I lead a very busy life. And I don't cook. But on the Skinny Chicks programme, you don't have to eat at home every night or follow an elaborate diet plan that makes you give up in a week. By understanding the sugar balance and the protein/carb combo, I can eat out every day if I so choose. Just knowing that I can eat at a fast-food Mexican restaurant or a five-star restaurant and not worry that I'm 'cheating' or off-track makes this one of the easiest weight-loss plans around.

But the real reason that I feel comfortable recommending this diet to patients who ask me about weight loss is its nutritional value. By following the Skinny Chicks programme, you're actually getting good nutrition and the vitamins and minerals your body needs for healthy living.

Dr Julie Edween
Los Angeles, California
Plastic Surgery Expert on the Discovery Channel's Plastic Surgery Beverly Hills *and The Learning Channel's* Bodywork

Dr Julie Edween is a board-certified facial plastic and cosmetic surgeon. She received her medical degree and graduated as Magna Cum Laude from Kansas City University of Medicine and Biosciences and was trained in Facial Plastic Surgery at Michigan State University Botsford Hospital. She then completed a cosmetic fellowship through the American Academy of Cosmetic Surgery in Southern California.

Introduction

Are you one of those people whose idea of dieting is starving yourself all day – and then stuffing yourself with a great big salad at night? Have you tried this approach and been happy with the results? Of course not. Because without ever having met you, I know that even if you lost weight in the short term, you put it all back on. We just can't live on salad alone.

I know, because I've been there myself. The Skinny Chicks programme came out of my own need to get off the diet merry-go-round, to get fit and healthy and stop making myself crazy with food. I lived the life of eating salads during the day and bingeing on sweets at night. I guinea-pigged my way through every diet gimmick there was. I cycled through all the major diets: the Atkins diet, the grapefruit diet, the cabbage soup diet, the Mayo Clinic diet, the Sugar Busters diet, to name a few. I tried over-the-counter supplements and diet aids, Chinese herbs and, at one point during my twenties, I even stooped to stealing my grandfather's prescription Lasix (a diuretic) to lose weight. When that didn't work, I paid someone to hypnotize me so I could get my eating under control. Needless to say, that didn't work either – and it was expensive too! I didn't know or care whether I lost water weight, muscle tissue or fat. I only cared about making the numbers on the scales go down.

After I had exhausted every possible fad diet and weight loss trick, I finally gave up and looked up. I prayed for God to point me in the proper direction. Then I met a nutritionist who suggested I learn more about food and the body if I really wanted to understand how to lose weight. As many of my clients do today, I argued with my nutritionist. I was very emotional about food, and I wanted to cling to my habits. I basically wanted her seal of approval for my existing ways. It took a lot of persuasion for me to let go of the low-carb concept. But eventually I realized that even though my background was in modelling, fitness and personal training, I didn't fundamentally understand what was preventing me from losing weight. I decided to train as a nutritionist, and there I found the answer to my prayers.

I learned that eating too little food would slow down my metabolism more and more; that eating too much would cause fat storage; and finally that eating to keep blood sugar levels stable was the key to avoiding sugar cravings and thus putting the weight back on.

It was difficult for me to accept these concepts. All I wanted to do was restrict carbs and calories and watch the scales magically go down 10 pounds in a week, as they had so many times before.

But somehow, it all finally clicked. I started to eat balanced meals such as low-fat cottage cheese mixed with fresh fruit and yogurt, topped with crunchy walnuts; banana–peanut butter smoothies; and pumpkin pancakes (all of these recipes are in this book), and I went from an American size 12 to a size 5 (UK size 14 to a size 8) in 3 months. Best of all I was eating real food, not diet food, and those insatiable cravings for sweets and salty carbs were virtually eliminated. I was so excited to be 'freed' from the bondage of 'dieting' that I vowed to get this message to all the people who were suffering just like me. It was one of the best things that ever happened to me.

By eating the Skinny Chicks way, you *will* lose weight – anywhere from 2 to 8 pounds (0.9 to 3.6 kilograms) in the first 2 weeks alone – and you'll notice an improvement in your moods and overall outlook on life as well.

What's so great about this weight loss plan is that it is not a diet – it is an *eating plan*. I will teach you some basic body science principles regarding weight loss that will resonate with you the moment you read them. On my eating plan, you will learn how to programme your metabolism to burn fat and save muscle 24 hours a day. Most people on this plan first notice weight loss in their mid-section; then they notice an increase in energy and a happier mood, usually within the first week. Even better, you will not feel deprived or undernourished. You will never starve yourself because you'll be eating four or even five fully balanced meals a day (that's right, I said four or five meals a day, not three meals and two snacks). In fact, you might be tempted to say, as did one Skinny Chick client of mine, 'Are you sure this isn't a gain-weight pro-gramme?' I promised her, and I promise you, it's not.

The Skinny Chicks programme is for people who have real lives and live in the real world, with jobs, families and other responsibilities. My nutrition plan works for today's fast-paced lifestyle. I've included fast-food meals, high-end restaurant meals and delicious, healthy recipes you can cook for yourself and your family. I've also included more than 60 quick 'grab and go' meals – great for students and busy working mums alike.

You're going to eat normal meals. You don't cut out carbs, you don't cut out fats, you don't cut out sugar. You can have desserts. You won't be eating boiled chicken and steamed broccoli at every meal. And best of all, you won't be eating salads for dinner.

The Skinny Chicks plan is the healthiest way to lose weight and keep it off. You don't have to starve yourself (in fact, you'll be defeating your dieting goals if you do). You don't have to weigh and measure your food. You don't have to cut out carbs. You don't have to be perfect. You can have pasta. You can even have sweets and crisps (I'll tell you which ones are best and how and when to eat them). You can exercise a moderate amount and get the benefits you need. If you want to eat a salad, be my guest – I'll tell you how to make it properly. In other words, you can live in the real world and still lose weight. I know, because that's the life I live. And I love it.

My goal is to explain it to you so that it's easy, so that it makes sense, and so that you'll really understand how the food you eat will affect your body and your life. I'm going to lay it out in a way that will change the way you eat for ever.

So put down the salad fork and get ready to enjoy eating again. Before you know it, you'll be a Skinny Chick just like the hundreds and hundreds of clients I've helped with my Skinny Chicks programme. You have nothing to lose but your cravings!

PART I

SKINNY CHICKS

LEARN THE

SCIENCE

CHAPTER 1

How Salads Got Us into Big Fat Trouble

4 a.m. on a Tuesday

I roll my puffy body off the edge of my warm, fluffy pillow-top bed. I'm suffering from a 'food hangover'. Why? Because last night, while discussing the ex-boyfriend with my beloved Aunt Sandra, I munched through an entire box of Ritz biscuits, a bag of marshmallows, and a jar of peanut butter. Now I'm bloated from all that sodium and feel like a huge brick is sitting in my lower stomach.

So I do what I do every morning: gulp down two pots of coffee. Not two cups, two *pots*. That's why I need to wake up so very early; I need enough time to drink the coffee and visit the toilet several times before heading to the gym to teach my hour-long Spinning class. Of course, I skip breakfast – I have to make up for all the calories consumed during last night's biscuit–peanut butter–marshmallow sandwich binge.

I go to the gym and teach my Spin class, and work out as hard as I can.

8.30 a.m.

After class I'm famished and shaking because my blood sugar is so low. I'm so angry about bingeing last night, though, that I decide to skip breakfast, resist my hunger and head home to take a shower. Afterwards,

I go down into the kitchen to prepare the lunch I'll take to the office: a BIG salad. It has to be BIG because I'm starving like an abandoned kitten and I still have hours to go before lunchtime, so I use a whole head of iceberg lettuce, a pepper, half a cucumber, three sticks of celery, one large beefsteak tomato, one head of broccoli, one head of cauliflower, artichoke hearts (tinned in water, not oil, of course), alfalfa sprouts and half a bottle of low-cal salad dressing.

1 p.m.

Nine hours after waking up, I'm finally ready to eat my first meal. At this point, I am really forgetful, agitated and feeling so shaky I can barely remember my own name. I am so excited to take my first bite, because (a) it's healthier than what I ate last night and (b) I'm finally on the right track with my eating! Now I'm sure to lose weight.

3 p.m.

I'm still full from my lunch salad and I feel pretty good. And yet . . . I feel like I *need* to have something sweet. I find myself fantasizing about a chocolate chip cookie; don't I deserve at *least* one? After all, I've been awake since 4 a.m., I worked out like a banshee and the only thing I've eaten all day is a salad! How much damage can one cookie do? I'm going for that cookie and then – I promise – I will get back on track.

3.30 p.m.

At the deli, my special chocolate chip cookie is warm, soft, moist and smells like fresh-baked heaven. I love it. I *need* it. Hey – it's gone already! That wasn't even close to enough. I buy a mini lemon cake (it's made with fruit, so it must be healthy) and as I devour it, the battle inside my head begins:

> *Christine . . . what the **** are you doing? This is not on your diet. You're such a loser, you can't even resist sweets for less than 24 hours.*
> *Your diet is shot.*
> *So what? Fine. I'm a loser. Who cares!*

I buy two more mini lemon cakes and four more chocolate chip cookies and sneak them back to the office in my handbag. I eat them all within 2 hours, keeping the door to my office – where I work as the aerobics manager of a popular health club – closed.

10 p.m.

I decided not to eat dinner because I had so many calories during my afternoon diet meltdown. At around 10 p.m., I have a small serving of low-fat frozen yogurt, reckoning that that must be OK since I haven't had dinner. I decide I can have a second serving because the first one was so small, and this time I add some caramel syrup. (The caramel syrup bottle reads 'fat free', after all.) The rest of the evening continues with more sweets, and I honestly can't stop myself. More than I crave love, companionship or any emotional need – I crave sugar. The more I eat, the more I crave. These are not subtle cravings; they rule my every thought as well as my actions. Sugar is my significant other – like a toxic boyfriend that I can't break up with.

As I down these treats, I carry on a running argument with myself: *Am I a sugar addict? How can I be, when I'm so good that I exercise, skip meals and eat only salad?* I want to sleep, but I'm so wired from all the sugar that I can't turn off the voices in my head.

I am completely out of control.

What I didn't realize was that I craved sugar because I basically fasted for the first 9 hours of my day. I had convinced myself that if I skipped breakfast, ate a BIG salad for lunch, skipped dinner and ate 'just a few' sweets during the day, I would finally lose weight. I kept this up for several years. It may have been a twisted way of thinking, but it was my reality.

And that is how salads got me into big fat trouble. I believe this is how salads get lots of girls into big fat trouble. Guys don't do this . . . it's only girls who eat this way and convince ourselves that it's 'low-calorie eating'. When we see slim women eating 'real' food, we think to ourselves, 'Oh, she has a special blessing from God, and that's why she can eat normal meals and I'm stuck with eating rabbit food.' Let me be the first to tell you that you *can* eat 'normal' food and be thin, too.

Skinny Chick 10-Week Transformation

NAME: JULIA S.

AGE: 34

TOTAL POUNDS LOST: 27¼ (12.4 kg)

TOTAL INCHES LOST: 31½ (80 cm)

I started putting on weight about 4 years ago, and each year it seemed like I put on more than the year before. This was a big change for me. As a child, I was very active. I played a lot of sports, and I never had a problem with food. My family is very health conscious. We all exercise and eat well. So I could not work out out why I was gaining this weight.

Part of it was definitely my social lifestyle. I was drinking and partying and hanging out late at night, and I got a little carried away. I wasn't organizing my time properly. When partying and eating and drinking became a priority, I knew I had to back off.

Christine helped me change some bad habits. I now have breakfast every day, something I never did before. I learned to combine proteins with carbs. And, of course, I learned that skinny girls don't eat salads. I used to say, 'I'm watching my weight, I'll just eat a salad'. I realize that doesn't work. But if I have a nice *healthy* salad, with a little chicken or some egg white, I feel better and can stick to my goals. I've learned to enjoy foods that are healthy. Double bacon cheeseburgers are great, but they're not giving my body the nutrition it needs.

Life can be so overwhelming, and sometimes it feels you're just living day to day, trying to make it, not really achieving the things you set out to do. Now, with the Skinny Chicks programme, I know that once I put my mind to doing something, I *can* do it. I feel inspired to let the real Julia come out and shine. I look back and see that all my fat was covering so much beauty. Can I just pat myself on the back?

It all starts with stepping away from the salad mentality and learning the truth about what makes us crave what we shouldn't eat and why eating what we shouldn't is so bad for us.

Why Skinny Chicks Don't Eat Salads

Back in 1999, I was 2 stone 2 pounds (13.6 kilograms) overweight, and it seemed like nothing could help me lose the excess (more than 2 stone). Now, after learning about how food works in the body, I am in the best shape of my life. I've come to realize that weight loss is not accomplished through a fad diet or TV exercise gimmick; it is a matter first and foremost of the heart. Once your heart is on board, it is a matter of educating yourself about sensible nutrition.

One day, two friends and I were dining at a popular restaurant. Deep in conversation, I didn't take time to study the menu carefully, and when the waiter asked for my order, I just went with a salad. As is often the case, my two friends echoed my order, assuming that I – a nutritionist – had made a healthy choice. When our meals arrived, all three of us looked at the salads and back at each other . . . and burst out laughing. They looked like erupting volcanoes, massive piles of breaded chicken strips and chunks of three different kinds of cheese, all smothered in a creamy dressing.

We were embarrassed by the sheer quantity of food in front of us. The salads were not only unhealthy, they were definitely *not* conducive to losing weight. In fact, these 'healthy' dishes probably contained more than 1,000 calories! I told my friends that anybody 'dieting' on these salads would become obese within weeks, and then blurted out, 'I'll tell you one thing . . . skinny chicks don't eat salads!'

We think of salads as a very light meal (as opposed to a big steak or a plate of lasagne) and, indeed, half an iceberg lettuce contains only about 39 calories, with trace amounts of vitamins and no fat. No wonder most people believe that eating salad is a healthy alternative to high-calorie foods and a basic building block of any weight loss plan.

But when it comes to nutrition and weight loss, all salads are not created equal. For our grandparents, a salad usually consisted of lettuce, tomatoes and cucumbers, drizzled with a bit of vinegar and olive oil. Have you watched a cooking programme lately? Or eaten in a restaurant? Everything comes super-sized with a list of ingredients that takes up half the menu page.

Nowadays, when you order a salad from any restaurant, be it a fast-food place or an expensive eatery, you are going to get a huge amount of lettuce topped with two or three kinds of cheese, perhaps pecans or slivered almonds, breaded and fried chicken, bacon bits or dried cranberries and buttery fried croutons – all drenched with calorie-laden dressing.

After the volcano salad incident, I decided to do a little field research. I ordered salads from several popular restaurants and got them to pack every ingredient separately. I weighed all the individual toppings, plugged them into my food database and added up the calories in each salad. What I found out was that there were actually more calories in a Cobb salad (a garden salad including iceberg lettuce, tomato, bacon, chicken breast, hard-boiled egg, avocado and Roquefort cheese) than an icing-smothered Cinnabon (a highly calorific American cinnamon bun)! The results were so unbelievable – shocking in fact – that *E! News* did a story on them.

SALADS	CALORIES	FAT (G)	CARB (G)	PROTEIN (G)
Cheesecake Factory Caesar Salad	1,699	145	44	65
Applebee's Stacked Tostada Salad	1,409	119	38	50
Cheesecake Factory Cobb Salad	1,340	96	47	74
Applebee's Oriental Chicken Salad	1,237	74	91	58
Chili's Southwestern Cobb Salad	1,117	82	40	56
Macaroni Grill Chicken Caesar Salad	675	44	14	50

Note: all US statistics

By contrast, here are some fast foods that we would never dare touch while dieting, yet actually contain fewer calories than the typical restaurant salad.

FAST FOODS	CALORIES	FAT (G)	CARB (G)	PROTEIN (G)
Burger King Whopper	678	37	53	31
In-N-Out Double Double with Cheese	670	41	40	37
McDonald's Big Mac with Cheese	563	32	43	25
Dairy Queen Double Homestyle Cheeseburger	540	31	30	35
Taco Bell Seven Layer Burrito	530	22	67	18
Wendy's Double Cheeseburger	458	25	34	25
Taco Bell Double Decker Supreme	380	18	40	15

Note: all US statistics

Of course, a small salad with a little bit of dressing before or after a meal is just fine. But substituting a salad for a more diverse variety of healthy and satisfying foods, and then filling up with sugary treats as a reward for that 'sacrifice', causes erratic blood sugar levels – just the opposite of what we need to lose weight.

The Key to Losing Weight

Before we go on, I'd like you to take a short quiz. Which of these symptoms have you experienced in the past 2 weeks?

- Headaches
- Sugar cravings
- Caffeine cravings
- Shakiness/dizziness
- Mood swings/irritability
- Lethargy/lack of energy
- Lack of concentration
- Extreme hunger

Skinny Chick 10-Week Transformation

NAME: Jessica C.
AGE: 29
TOTAL POUNDS LOST: 27 (12.2 kg)
TOTAL INCHES LOST: 27½ (70 cm)

I've been overweight since about the age of 6 or 7. I was a latchkey kid growing up, and I didn't have much adult supervision in the morning or afternoon. When I got home from school, I did what kids normally do: eat junk food and watch TV. I lived on instant noodles, peanut butter and Doritos. When you're a kid, you don't know any better; you just go with what tastes good. Then I went to university and the problem got even worse because I had free rein with junk food.

When I was 20 years old, my mother's sister passed away from complications of obesity. She was only 50 years old. She was diabetic and had had a lot of health issues that come from being overweight. That was a wake-up call for me, and it made me take a look at my life. I began to eat better and make better choices, and I tried to exercise more. It helped a lot. I went from a US size 24 (UK size 26) to about a US size 18 (UK size 20). For somebody who weighed about 18 stone (114 kilograms), that was a big difference. But then I stopped losing weight.

I tried a lot of different diets, none of which really worked. I tried the Zone diet; just not eating; and even a crazy diet that was supposed to take off 10 pounds (4½ kilograms) in 3 days. No surprise, it didn't work. After those 3 days, you lose about 5 pounds (2¼ kilograms), but you're so demoralized and hungry that you put about 7 pounds (3.2 kilograms) back on. All the diets I tried were too hard to follow, and they didn't really let you live your life.

And *all* of these diets tell you to have meals made of salads. To make your salad have more pizzazz, you keep throwing vegetables in there.

You start to hate vegetables, which makes it even worse. At the end of the day, you eat the same thing every day and you just hate it all.

A year and a half ago I got engaged, and ever since then I've been even more focused on losing weight. Each time I start a new diet, I stick to it for about a month and then life gets in the way. Now that I'm planning a wedding, I have a lot to do and no time for diets that require a lot of cooking, a lot of different ingredients or just a lot of sacrifice.

And then the Skinny Chicks programme came along. It allowed me to live my life – and I've now lost nearly a stone (13 kilograms) and gone down several sizes.

Even if I weren't getting married, I would love this programme because it's a life change, not just a temporary thing. It's easy to follow. It doesn't require any cooking skills, no secret formula, no counting points. It's flexible, too. It's easy to estimate your portions so you don't have to weigh and measure everything. You just listen to your body. If you're really hungry, then you may have a little bit more. It's not rocket science.

This is a way of life I can continue to follow. What greater gift than to know you can have good health for ever? It doesn't get much better than that.

If you ticked several items on the list, you are riding the blood sugar roller-coaster, a cycle that will have you feeling cheerful one minute and down in the dumps the next . . . not to mention overtired, overwhelmed and overweight.

What if I were to tell you that keeping your blood sugar on a healthy, even keel would help you get rid of these annoying and debilitating symptoms without starvation or deprivation – and help you lose weight in the process? All you have to do is make a few simple, non-extreme dietary changes.

If you do occasionally experience the symptoms above, don't hit the panic button. It just means you haven't eaten for a while and your brain cells need a little fuel. Where do they get that fuel? From the carbohydrates you eat (so much for the 'healthy' no-carb diet).

In this book, I'll explain the basics of blood sugar, what it does in your body, and why keeping blood sugar levels stable is the single most important concept in losing weight. It also increases your energy and has a host of other benefits. So, if you take away just one principle from this book, let it be this: *The key to losing weight and keeping it off is keeping your blood sugar stable.* Understand this concept, apply it to how and what you eat, and it will be transformative.

What Is Blood Sugar, Anyway?

Blood sugar (glucose) is by no means a bad thing. In fact, our bodies need glucose to function; it's the primary fuel that our cells use. Some cells, such as brain, nerve and red blood cells, can run only on glucose. Your blood sugar level refers to the amount of glucose in your blood.

As I said before, glucose comes from the carbohydrates we eat. When most people think of carbs, they automatically think of french fries, white bread, rice, pasta, and sweets like cakes and doughnuts. But veggies, whole grains, fruits and beans are also packed with carbs – and in fact, they're the best sources of carbs. Here's another important factoid to remember: whether the carbs you eat come from pasta, rice or grains, no matter how much you eat at one sitting, your brain cells will need more carbs 4 hours later. The brain and nervous system don't store glucose. When glucose levels are low, the body begins to break down liver and muscle glycogen (glucose) for fuel. So, no new carbs, no fresh fuel for brain cells and the body begins to break down its own tissues – thus the head-ache you get when you eat a late lunch. Carbs get a bad rap. A huge industry has sprung up around the notion that carbs are evil. (Witness the shelves at the supermarket; they're stocked with no-carb and low-carb products.) How can something your body needs to function, to run its own command centre – your brain – be bad for you? Simply put, they're not. As a nutritionist, I get into a lot of confrontations with bright people who are convinced they need to cut out carbs to lose weight. The reality is that you *need* carbs every 4 hours. But the trick is getting the right amount of the right carbs at the right times. In this book, you'll learn how many carbs you really need to eat, what you need to eat them with and the best times to eat them. And, as you'll find out, it's as easy as ABC.

In the next chapters, I'll explain the principles behind the Skinny Chicks programme and why it will work for you. You'll hear from real people how this programme works in the real world through testimonials from some of my private practice clients as well as from some participants in the Skinny Chicks test group. When I started to write this book, I wanted to be sure that the programme I developed would be just as effective as the individualized plans I create for my private clients, so I invited a group of people to go on the Skinny Chicks journey with me. Twenty intrepid women followed the programme in this book for 10 weeks, kept journals and answered weekly questionnaires. The group lost a combined total of 21 stone 6 pounds (140 kilograms), an average of 15½ pounds (7 kilograms) per person, 23 inches (58 centimetres) per person and a total of 452 inches (1,148 centimetres) lost over 10 weeks! It was more successful than even I imagined. You'll meet some of these people throughout the book and hear their stories.

One important thing that came out of this group is that the Skinny Chicks programme is redefining skinny. It's no longer the rail-thin, 'I only eat lettuce' model. If a size 12 is skinny for you, that's great. For someone else, it might be a size 4. You're skinny when you're empow-ered with knowledge, when your blood sugar is balanced and when you live a healthy lifestyle.

CHAPTER 2

The ABCs of Weight Loss

Nutrition isn't simple. As with so many things in life, moderation is the key. If you take any nutritional solution too far, it doesn't work. The perfect example is eating zero carbs. Yes, you will lose weight because the body will eventually break down body fat for energy. There are only a couple of snags: (1) it may promote the development of kidney stones, cause acidosis (increase the acidity of the body's fluids), decrease calcium balance and increase the risk of bone loss; and (2) most of us will end up crawling into the kitchen in the middle of the night to get our hands on the stuff our brains need: cakes, biscuits, doughnuts, ice cream, anything with carbs in it. This is no way to live a happy life. Here's the thing: you don't have to give up carbs to live a happy life. You don't have to become a 'slave to the crave' that hits you when your blood sugar is out of kilter.

Your blood sugar starts out on the low side in the morning because while you sleep, you essentially fast for 7 to 8 hours or more. Your Skinny Chicks goal is to keep your blood sugar stabilized, which is defined as anywhere between 80 and 120 milligrams of glucose per decilitre of blood. Anywhere above or below this range can result in fat storage, as indicated by the unhappy faces in the chart on page 15.

ERRATIC BLOOD SUGAR

If you are like me, you are a busy woman and you don't always have time to eat breakfast. Most of us consider that to be a good thing because we actually think that starving ourselves is the way to lose weight. But take a look at the chart above and see what happens to blood sugar levels on a typical day for a typical salad eater.

Now, remember that brain cells can only function with glucose for fuel, and since the body doesn't store it in a readily accessible state, you need to give it more approximately every 4 hours. This applies to every human being alive. When you wake up in the morning and you haven't eaten for 8 hours or more, your body has already dipped into your reserve fuel storage (glycogen from your liver and muscle tissues – more on that later) and the tank is empty.

When we break down and succumb to that morning sugary coffee drink or Danish pastry, our blood sugar shoots from super low to super high. Hunger goes away but returns quickly as blood sugar rapidly drops, leaving us hungrier than ever for 'real food'. Once we finally eat our big salad, we have a little – but not nearly enough – of what our body needs: carbs. Throughout the rest of the day, we are essentially miserable and on a constant lookout for a little treat. Remember, the brain has barely had its required glucose all day. At night, the need for fuel is stronger than our willpower could ever be, so we cave in and eat sweets like Miss Piggy on a breakup binge.

What happens when you drink that sugary coffee or eat a bag of sweets on an empty stomach? Your body gets flooded with glucose, which causes your pancreas to release large amounts of insulin to carry the glucose to the cells for fuel. This puts us in a hyperglycaemic (spiked blood sugar) state, and if there is more glucose than our cells can use, the extra calories are stored as fat. Insulin does the job of clearing away blood glucose extremely well, and soon blood sugar levels are low again. That's when you find yourself feeling hungry again an hour or two later.

The Insulin/Blood Sugar Connection

As you can see from the chart on page 15, your blood sugar levels are influenced by what you eat and when you eat it. You've probably heard of insulin and blood sugar levels before, but you may have thought they were only important to people with diabetes. Actually, we should all be concerned about blood sugar, especially those of us who are trying to lose weight.

The easiest way to understand the way the glucose/insulin process works is to think of insulin as a parcel delivery system. I like to call it FatEx. Inside the FatEx delivery van are parcels of glucose. The van travels around in the interstitial fluid of the body (the fluid that is found in between cells), pulls up to a cell, knocks on the door and says, 'Hi, I'm here to deliver a parcel.' The cell door opens up, accepts the parcel and gets its glucose delivery. The FatEx van then continues on its route and travels around to the next cell. Sometimes the cell door doesn't open; the response is, 'Oh no, we don't need a parcel of glucose right now, we have enough. Go to a different cell.' So the little FatEx van keeps on driving around to all the cells, and eventually the cells become 'insulin resistant' and stop accepting glucose.

When that happens, the insulin FatEx van is forced to circulate around in the bloodstream and in between cells until finally the body says, 'Enough. We don't have room for any more parcels.' What does anyone do when they run out of room? They put the leftovers in storage units. The body's storage space is the fat cell. At this point, the conversion of glucose to fatty acids is accomplished by insulin's activation of several enzymes, especially one called lipoprotein lipase. When that happens, the FatEx van leaves a special rush delivery on your rear end and parks itself on your hips!

The point is that although you need carbs every 4 hours, you don't want to flood your system with glucose by eating too many carbs at one time. But you also don't want to deprive your system of glucose by eating too *few* carbs.

Let's take a look at a stable blood sugar chart below. Here we have a balanced meal that includes protein, carbs and healthy fats, eaten within 1 hour of waking up. This is followed by another small, balanced meal every 4 hours throughout the day. The result? Blood sugar levels that are

STABILIZED BLOOD SUGAR

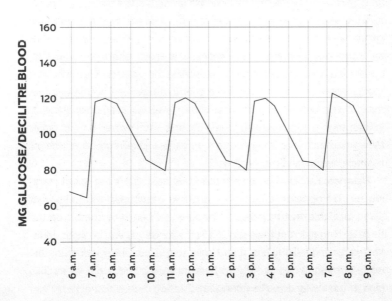

never too high and never too low. This is the optimal condition for fat burning because your body draws energy from blood sugar (from food) and fat storage. What's more, you have steady energy and stable hormones (more on these in Chapter 3) *and* you aren't starving to death.

As Easy as A, B, C and D

Understanding blood sugar, hormonal responses, fat storage and fat burning in your body is one thing, but actually making it work in your real life so that you can lose weight is another thing entirely. That is why I break it down into ABC & D: Amount, Balance, Clock and Darnit, Get Your Lazy Butt on the Treadmill. Each of these is explained in detail in subsequent chapters, but here they are in a nutshell.

Amount: Many people think that dieting means eating less. But the truth is, slashing calories alone will not help you lose weight. Let me explain. When you skip breakfast or any other meal, you slow your resting metabolic rate – the number of calories your body burns at rest. Metabolism is the process whereby the body converts food into energy, uses it for repairs or stores it as fat for future use. In simple terms, a faster metabolism burns calories more efficiently and stores less fat. A slower metabolism burns calories less efficiently and therefore causes more calories to be stored as fat. When insufficient food is present in the stomach, ghrelin levels are high (ghrelin is a hormone, produced by cells lining the stomach, that stimulates the appetite). Ghrelin levels increase prior to a meal and decrease after a meal. If you don't eat enough, your ghrelin levels will keep poking at your insides, saying, 'Feed me! Feed me!' Chapter 3 will explain how to determine how much food you need to satisfy these ghrelin gremlins, lose (or maintain) weight and stay healthy.

Balance: Eating to keep your blood sugar stable is not about starving; just the opposite. On the Skinny Chicks eating plan you can have it all. In fact, the key to success is having it *all at once* by combining the three leading macronutrients found in the foods you eat: proteins, high-fibre carbs and healthy fats. If you want to give your body optimum fuel while burning fat, you've got to balance your blood sugar levels. Too high or too low and you're storing fat or losing muscle tissue. I'll tell you exactly what you need to eat – and when – in order to stabilize your blood sugar, save muscle and, most importantly, burn fat. When you read Chapter 4, you will learn a diet principle so easy and so logical, you will wonder why you never knew it before. And when you put it into practice, you will wish you had known it a long time ago.

Keeping balance in the body is vitally important. Think about what happens when you drink wine on an empty stomach. It goes 'straight to your head'. It is absorbed into your bloodstream very quickly and delivered directly to your brain. However, if you eat something along with the wine, it slows down the delivery to the brain. The same thing happens when you sit down at a restaurant, ravenously hungry and start eating bread before dinner. Bread on an empty stomach is absorbed into the bloodstream very quickly, causing your blood sugar level to spike. The trick in Chapter 4 will help you slow down this process and sustain your energy throughout the day.

Clock: The symptoms listed in the quiz in Chapter 1 appear most commonly when you've waited too long between meals. The Skinny Chicks programme recommends that you eat every 4 hours. That's because your brain and nervous system can store only enough glucose to fuel them for about 4 hours. After that, they go for the stored glycogen (the main form in which glucose is stored in the body) in your liver and muscle tissue. And when you break down liver and muscle tissue, *you dramatically slow down metabolism.* In simple terms, if you go too long without food, your body thinks there is a food shortage and your metabolism tends to slow down. Meals eaten too far apart promote fat storage, low energy, headaches and sugar cravings.

'Darnit, Get Your Lazy Butt on the Treadmill': We all lose muscle mass as we get older. We can also lose muscle mass from lack of use. Muscle cells are about eight times more metabolically demanding than fat cells, so the greater your proportion of muscle to fat, the faster your metabolic rate will be.

Eating decent-sized meals every 4 hours was a dream come true for a body-image-obsessed girl like me. And eating delicious meals such as Cinnamon raisin oaty muffins; pasta with meat sauce; grilled chicken breast sandwiches; or cheese with fruit and wine? That doesn't sound like diet food because it's *not*. The Skinny Chicks plan isn't about depriving and starving; it's about giving your body what it really needs, when it needs it.

DON'T IGNORE YOUR ABCs

The silliest thing is that the ABCs are all naturally built into every human being – we just ignore them. If you are a parent, you know that a newborn baby needs food every few hours. Toddlers are constantly hungry and ask for food when they need it. They don't care if it's 'time' for a meal or not; they just know their bodies need fuel. Adults learn to ignore hunger pangs if they're in the middle of an important work project, only to overeat several hours later when they finally get a chance to take a break. When they follow that pattern week after week, month after month, year after year, they end up in my office complaining that they are fat even though they eat healthily. Surprisingly, most clients come to me with the same story. It goes something like this: 'In my school and university years I could eat whatever I wanted and never put on weight, but now I just have to look at food and I pile on the pounds.' Then they blame it on their age. But the truth is, they are putting on weight now because all those days of skipping meals have caused their metabolisms to slow to a crawl – so that their bodies cling to every calorie they *do* eat.

Meet Giuliana, Who Woke Up Run Down

Giuliana Rancic was on top of the world. She had met the love of her life and landed her dream job as the host of *E! News* on the E! Network. Life was good! So why did she feel so awful? She was exhausted all the time. She had absolutely no energy and was downright irritable. Plus, she had put on about 10 pounds (4½ kilograms). That might not seem like much, but for a girl as small as Giuliana, the extra weight added up to her not being able to fit into her clothes. (Not to mention that every day, her weight gain was reflected back to her plus 10 pounds on television.) Instead of waking up in the morning filled with excitement and anticipation, she woke up feeling sad and run down. She didn't know it at the time, but her weariness and malaise were the result of her unhealthy eating habits. Here is her story.

> *Most days I was so busy at work that I didn't make time to eat. On a typical day I would skip breakfast and lunch. By dinnertime I was so famished I would eat not one, but two dinners – I had to make up for the meals I skipped during the day, didn't I? I would hardly finish stuffing myself before my sweet tooth started calling. Why shouldn't I have a bowl of frozen yogurt, or a whole tub even? I had hardly eaten all day. The morning after a sugar binge, I would wake up feeling like I had a hangover. Not to mention the emotional hangover – I was so full of shame and so angry at myself that I'd swear off food for the whole day only to repeat the cycle at night when I got home.*

> *I bought every diet book on the market; I spent hours on the Internet searching for advice, but nothing helped. I was depressed and at my wit's end. That's when I turned to Christine for help. The first time I met Christine, she explained to me that my eating habits were causing blood sugar levels to spike then dip. She clued me in to the fact that the way I was eating was causing my uncontrollable sugar cravings and that my blood sugar ups and downs were actually the reason for my weight gain and my inability to lose weight. Right then and there, I signed up for her programme, and I haven't turned back. At first I thought it was willpower that was behind my ability to put the brakes on my nightly sugar binges, then I realized the reality was that I hadn't conquered my cravings, I had stopped having them! Christine's programme enabled me to lose the weight, but even more importantly, I now wake up in the morning feeling excited about my day.*

There's No Need to Be Hungry

Like Giuliana, many of us are confused by all the diet info out there, and this lack of knowledge can severely affect our quality of life, for a lifetime! We try this diet and that, but ultimately we go back to our old

Skinny Chick 10-Week Transformation

NAME: RUTH W.
AGE: 39
TOTAL POUNDS LOST: 15 (6.8 kg)
TOTAL INCHES LOST: 18.5 (47 cm)

I was pretty slim as a child and up to the age of about 24. After my first child, I lost all the baby fat. But after the second, I didn't. I just kept putting on weight. I didn't really notice that I was putting it on until my husband started to notice. He still loves me, but it affected our relationship. I tried diet pills; I tried exercise. Nothing was working. I never imagined that eating more could actually help me lose weight. I was sceptical. I thought, is this a get-fat plan? But this morning my husband said, 'I want to thank Christine because you look hot!'

I learned that it is very important to look at the labels on everything you buy. I've reduced the amount of fat in my diet. I'm Latin, and I've learned how to cook fat-free Mexican food. I learned how to cook a lot of things that are low-calorie, home-made. I stopped eating out so much. I cook for a few hours on Sunday night after the baby is asleep. During the week, I can make 10 meals out of the chicken or fish I cooked on Sunday. It's inspired me to cook healthy meals for my whole family. My husband is actually losing weight on the programme too.

I'm definitely continuing with the programme. This programme changed the way that I eat. It's really improved my life. It's changed my health, the way I feel about myself. I love that I can eat. I love that I look great. I love that I am healthier. I just can't believe what this programme has done for me, for my body, for my health. It made me feel sexy again. It's changed my relationship with my husband. My husband is so grateful, and so am I.

barometer of weight loss success (or so we think): hunger. Nobody wants to feel hungry, but many of us girls do for some portion of each day. Most people on a diet see hunger as an accomplishment; it must be doing some good because it feels so bad. I know that's how I felt, and it's how many of my clients feel when they first come to my office. You don't have to feel that way any more. You can and should feel like a healthy, stable, empowered person who is capable of doing anything – not like someone who is weak, distracted by hunger and miserable.

CHAPTER 3

It's the Amount That Counts

When it comes to nutrition, health and weight loss, one of the topics that really gets me fired up is the idea that starving yourself will help you lose weight. My philosophy is that in order to lose weight, we should *not* be eating less; just the opposite – we should be eating *more*. One of the most important messages of this book is that you should never starve yourself. Skipping meals is what leads to overeating, and that's not a good thing.

I never want you to skip meals. In fact, as you'll soon see, I want you to *add* meals to your day. This is great news for everyone who loves to eat (and who doesn't?). But how much food should you be eating? How important is it to eat a healthy, balanced meal? To this day, there are many people in the health and fitness industry who say that it doesn't matter what you eat or when, and all that matters is the number of calories. These CICO (Calories In Calories Out) theorists believe that human nutrition is as simple as eat-more-weigh-more and eat-less-weigh-less. If you subscribe to this logic, the plan of skipping meals and centring your diet around big fat salads looks like a winning strategy, right? And it would work fine if it weren't for one small glitch: human physiology.

'I'm Starving, but I'm Losing Weight'

Just for the sake of argument, let's see what happens if you actually avoid food for, say, 24 hours. Somewhere around 24 hours after your last meal, your body enters a state known as ketosis. (This state can also be reached by eating only protein and no carbs for approximately 24 to 48 hours.) In this state, your body begins to break down fat for fuel. If you are stranded on a deserted island and you have some extra body fat, this might help you last longer than your skinny sisters. But in the real world, you are bombarded with food temptation all day every day. By the 24th hour, you are insatiably thirsty, you have a bad taste in your mouth and the breath of a dragon, you have a nonstop headache and you are moping around like a hound dog. But guess what? You will be burning fat.

Before you go and just stop eating, let's think about some other things. Your hair and skin will be getting no nutrients, so your face will start to look haggard and worn. Your hair requires protein; A, B and D vitamins; iron; and a variety of other nutrients, so starving on and off for as little as 6 months is likely to make your hair brittle, frizzy and damaged. It will take you a whole year to regrow healthy hair. I don't know about you, but that is pretty much enough to convince me that starvation is not the way to go.

A more important consideration is that your muscles – including the most important muscle, your heart – are being broken down for fuel. Your metabolism has been reduced to the slowest possible crawl; fat burning is minimized since you have nothing to 'eat' besides your own body.

The body consists of trillions of cells, and all day long, each one performs its little cellular processes. Each of these processes requires various nutrients, enzymes and compounds that come from the foods we eat. On a starvation diet, the cells just don't get what they need and bad things start to happen. Let's look at the implications listed in the chart on page 26.

As you can see, starvation is not the way to healthy weight loss. Even if you have an iron will, you are doing more harm to your body than good. If you are like most people, you will find that rather than fasting

BODY PART	WHAT HAPPENS	WHAT'S THE PROBLEM?
Bones	Weak bones, osteoporosis	Lack of calcium
Energy level	Anaemia (tired all the time)	Lack of vitamin E, vitamin K, folate, iron, zinc, vitamin B_6 or vitamin B_{12}
Eyes	Dark circles under eyes	Not enough iron
Gastrointestinal tract	Constipation	Lack of fibre
Hair	Depigmentation (grey hair), slow hair growth	Not enough protein
Hair	Hair loss	Not enough biotin, B_6, B_{12} or folate
Hair	Dry and brittle hair	Not enough iodine
Mouth	Bleeding gums	Not enough vitamin C
Mouth	Cracked lips; swollen, dark red tongue	Not enough vitamin B_2 (riboflavin)
Skin	Dry, scaly, old-looking skin	Not enough essential fatty acids, vitamin E or protein
Skin	Greasy skin	Not enough vitamin B_2 (riboflavin)
Soft tissues	Delayed wound healing	Not enough vitamin A, vitamin C or zinc

entirely, you are actually snacking throughout the day to feed your body's basic need for glucose, and then overeating at night.

Why does this happen? The answer is that your body uses regulatory and counter-regulatory hormones to balance the chemicals in your body. This is why dieters can get so ratty! Insulin, cortisol, epinephrine (adrenaline), ghrelin and leptin all play a role. Remember those ghrelin gremlins that are poking at your stomach, begging to be fed? When people say, 'she's hormonal', it's not just a phrase. Research studies have shown that the levels of these hormones in the bloodstream fluctuate greatly as a result of what we do – or don't – eat.

The 'OK, I'll Just Skip Breakfast' Myth

What about semi-starvation – just skipping a meal here or there? Let's see what happens then. Within 4 hours of any meal, your brain will once again be in need of fuel. The hormone ghrelin is released, causing hunger pangs. If you decide to 'be good' and skip a meal, your brain isn't just going to shut off; it will turn to reserve storage, taking sugar in the form of glycogen from the muscle and liver tissues. As soon as the brain has to go to these tissues for fuel, it is going to do two things: (1) slow down your metabolism because it thinks you are starving; and (2) start aching. Most people think they are unique in getting a headache when they skip lunch. The reality is that all human beings get lightheaded, headachy and all the other symptoms of hypoglycaemia when their blood sugar gets low.

Just as an illustration (the reality is a bit more complex), think of your body's fuel sources as reserve fuel tanks. We'll call them Tanks 1, 2, 3 and 4. Your body's Tank 1 is blood sugar energy from food. When you have recently eaten, your body is burning the least fat. When Tank 1 starts to get low (i.e. low blood sugar), your body dips into Tank 2 – glycogen stored in the liver and muscle tissues – along with some body fat. Once Tank 2 runs out, your body starts to consume its own muscles and vital protein tissues and fat (Tank 3). After a day or more of starving (or no carbs), your body will go into ketosis and actively use a lot of fat – Tank 4 – for energy.

The Skinny Chicks programme keeps you going between Tank 1 and Tank 2. I want you to use Tank 2 because that is where the fat burning occurs, but I want you to avoid Tank 3 because it means a slowed metabolism and loss of muscle – not to mention hunger, hypoglycaemia and pain.

	BODY'S PRIMARY FUEL SOURCE	TIME ELAPSED SINCE LAST MEAL	ARE YOU BURNING FAT?	RESULTS
Tank 1	Blood sugar (glucose from carbs)	None (immediate)	Yes, if eating correctly	Energy from 50% blood sugar and 50% fat – speeds up metabolism for optimal fat burning
Tank 2	Glycogen (glucose) stored in liver and muscles	3 to 5 hours	Yes, if eating correctly	
Tank 3	Muscles and vital tissues	5 to 6 hours or more	Yes – but ...	Dramatically slowed metabolism, consuming muscles
Tank 4	Body fat (ketosis)	24 to 72 hours	Yes – but ...	Dramatically slowed metabolism, very damaging to body and metabolism

Let's not take this 'slowed metabolism' thing lightly. Metabolism is commonly known as the breakdown of food inside the body and its transformation into energy. I define it as the sum of all the life processes of each of the trillions of cells in the body. With a faster metabolism, your body can burn more food, while a slower metabolism means that even when eating less, you can put on weight. When you eat the right amount at regular intervals, your body speeds up your metabolism. If your metabolism is faster, your body automatically burns fat all day and even at night when you are sleeping. When you starve yourself or skip a meal, your body thinks you're in a famine and it needs to help you survive. As Dr Lawrence Cheskin, of Johns Hopkins Weight Management Center in the US describes it, ' . . . when you're eating less for weight loss, your body begins to act as if it's being shortchanged. Your metabolism slows in an attempt to conserve fuel.' It will slow everything down so that it does not burn as many calories, including your rate of digestion, your circulation, your breathing and, of course, your brain

Skinny Chick Chat

DEAR CHRISTINE: I need to lose at least 1 stone 6 pounds (9 kilograms), and I've been eating one meal a day . . . if I can't lose weight on just one meal a day, how can I eat every 4 hours? You also mentioned that I would feel the symptoms of hypoglycaemia if I don't eat every 4 hours, but I've been a one-meal-a-day person for years, and I never feel the symptoms of hypoglycaemia. Can you tell me what is going on in my body?

SUZIE J.

SUZIE: You're what I call a 'body divorcée'. Don't feel bad; I hear this in my office quite often. When you first began skipping meals and/or waiting too long between meals, your body tried to nudge at you via the symptoms of hypoglycaemia. You say that you've been eating only one meal a day for a while, so you may not remember the subtle headaches, sugar cravings, depression and lack of concentration. But I guarantee you felt at least one if not more of the symptoms of hypoglycaemia when you first started skipping meals. The fact that you are not having those symptoms any longer is a sign of a severely damaged metabolism. Our relationships with our bodies can be compared with a marriage: In the beginning, the communication is very clear and blissful, but after several years of ignoring a nagging spouse, divorce (or at least estrangement) is the inevitable outcome. I believe our bodies are the same: your body tried to notify you not to wait too long between meals by giving you the warning signs of hypoglycaemia, but after years of trying to communicate with you, your body eventually gave up. Now you have zero communication and you don't feel the symptoms of hypoglycaemia. But take heart. Your body is very resilient and forgiving. Once you begin eating every 4 hours on a regular schedule, your body will open communication with you again, and you will be on the road to regaining a healthy metabolism. Try it and see for yourself!

EAT WELL, CHRISTINE

and nervous system functions. Then, when you have a late evening binge, your body can't burn the calories, and even small meals can result in fat storage. Metabolism is a hugely important concept in my programme.

Common Pitfalls for Dieters

I hope I have now convinced you that you shouldn't *ever* starve your-self. But this is not a licence to overeat at will. Overeating has become a huge problem in the West. The astonishing statistics say that around one in every four men and one in every three women in the UK are overweight; 24 per cent of women and 23 per cent of men are obese. Predictions from the UK Department of Health suggest that by 2010 around 6.6 million men and 6 million women in the UK will be obese. Everyone is worried about weight, either their own or their loved one's. The subject of nutrition used to be the ultimate wet blanket of cocktail party conversation, but now I find that everybody wants to talk to me about it. Even people who are in pretty good shape are wondering how they gain weight so easily.

What happens when we eat too much? What if, for instance, you ate a whole chocolate cake followed by a carrot cake chaser? (Unthinkable you say? Been there, done that. I ate whole cakes several times back in my salads and sweets days.) Even a less extreme example – say, following a large plate of pasta with an ice cream dessert – will trigger the same overeating effects. When you eat a huge helping of carbs, a load of glu-cose is dumped into your bloodstream all at once, causing your blood sugar levels to skyrocket. In reaction to the inundation of glucose, a fleet of insulin FatEx vans will be dispatched to deliver it. Only so much can be delivered to cells in need of fuel and to muscle and liver storage units; the rest will go into the one place that has an abundance of storage space: fat storage cells. This happens quickly (FatEx is very efficient), and before you know it, there is virtually no glucose left in your blood. It has literally gone from your lips to your hips. At that point, your blood sugar levels will take a nosedive – also not good. When levels fall too low, you get irritable and hungry very quickly, even if you've eaten only 2 hours before.

This is known as reactive hypoglycaemia. Your brain tells you to reach for more food, sweet food. Sugar-free food will not do; the body needs real glucose. You're very likely to give in to this sweet craving and reach for a doughnut or a few chocolate chip cookies, which will cause the cycle to repeat itself.

Most of us are not eating a whole chocolate cake at one sitting; more likely, it is a pastry from Starbucks on an empty stomach or a late night mini-binge of Häagen Dazs. But either way, this overeating is causing a small amount of fat storage each time.

So why is it that we are so much heavier than we were even 10 years ago? There are many different pieces of the puzzle. Some people blame the obesity epidemic on our sedentary lifestyles of computers, TV and video games. Yes, they are partially to blame. But to me, it's pure and simple: the reason is clearly our food intake. Portion sizes have increased in restaurants and fast-food outlets, and our knowledge of what constitutes a sensible portion has become distorted. Another problem is the inescapable presence of so many new, delicious food creations consisting of highly refined carbs and fats. You stroll down a supermarket aisle and see so many new biscuit and dessert innovations that you could eat a different one every night. You turn on the TV and you are lured to try the latest crispy/melty/gooey/cheesy/chocolatey/chewy products. It goes on and on. The common thread is usually a bleached flour–based carbohydrate or just a lot of sugar mixed with a large amount of fat (oil or butter). Fifteen years ago, most people had dinner and that was it. Now most people have dessert every night and a latte with a pastry at some point along the way.

The problem is that while your brain cells need carbs to function, your body can only handle a small amount of carbs at one time. So we need a strategy to make that fuel last longer and keep it from going into fat storage.

The best approach is not to starve yourself but to eat a reasonable amount at frequent intervals throughout the day. Not too much so that you overfeed your body's needs, but not too little so that you cause yourself to desire more later. The right amount of food (specifically, carbs) will elevate your blood sugar to an appropriate level, providing

Skinny Chick 10-Week Transformation

NAME: DIANNE M.
AGE: 31
TOTAL POUNDS LOST: 17½ (8 kg)
TOTAL INCHES LOST: 31¼ (79.4 cm)

I've always had a mental projection of myself as a 'big girl' ever since I was 9 years old and weighed about 7 stone (44 kilograms). Even when I was relatively small, my mental picture has always been of a big person who needed to cover herself up. The summer I was 9, my parents discovered wholesale stores and started buying sweets and chocolate bars in bulk. It made me feel really rich to be able to have this vast amount of food in my house. I really went out of control. When I started Year 5, I was a lot plumper than I had been the year before – and I stayed that way. At secondary school and university I relied on baggy shirts and men's jeans to hide my body.

For the past few years, I have basically had only one pair of trousers that I felt comfortable wearing: baggy combats that covered everything. Since following the Skinny Chicks programme, I have started to pull out things from my wardrobe, and now I'm fitting comfortably into US size 6 and size 8 (UK size 8 and 10) trousers; I've quadrupled my wardrobe options! I'm especially happy to have lost a lot of weight in my mid-section because I had a real problem with that 'muffin top' spilling out over my waistband.

I've tried other weight loss programmes where I felt like I was really suffering and restricting calories, but Christine's programme is special. I really like the way that Christine gave me a scientific programme and explained how combining carbs and proteins and essential fats in our diets helps our bodies work better and more efficiently. She gave us the tools to be able to eat for ever in a healthy way and not put on weight. I weighed and measured my food at the beginning of the programme, but I soon learned the portion sizes for my meals. Now I know exactly what 115 grams (4 ounces) of chicken looks like, and exactly what a portion of brown rice looks like. For me, the key to this programme is that you can do it with any food, in any place, at any supermarket, at any restaurant – not like other diets that make it difficult to go out into the world and live your real life.

I definitely feel healthier. I feel like my energy level has stabilized. When I started the programme, I had come from a place where I was feeling guilty about everything I put in my mouth. Now I feel like I have the tools to know exactly how my body is processing food and exactly what it requires, so I don't need to give it more and I don't need to give it less. Christine has shown me that you don't need to starve to get the body you want.

much-needed fuel for your brain and nervous system. If weight loss is the objective, you want to eat only enough to fuel the body's needs and no more, so there is no extra to be stored as fat. In this way, you actually feed your body all the nutrients it needs for energy, body function, immunity, skin, hair and hunger satiation, so that your muscles can do the work of burning calories from fat all day and night.

So, What Is a Reasonable Amount?

What seems like a reasonable amount of food to me may be something entirely different to you. There has to be some objective standard. That standard exists in the form of calories. A calorie is, basically, a unit of energy. Human beings function – breathe, move, digest, pump blood – on energy. The number of calories any food contains tells us how much potential energy is in that food. When we eat, metabolic processes burn the fuel and turn it into molecular substances that can be put to immediate use by our cells, or stored away as fat.

So, from the nutritional point of view, a reasonable amount of food is the number of calories your cells need to function well. That number is different for every person.

How Do You Determine How Many Calories to Eat?

I recommend eating a consistent number of calories at breakfast, lunch and dinner. As for snacks, you should be eating every 4 hours, so you may not need a mid-morning snack, depending on your schedule. However, for most people, the gap between lunch and dinner stretches well beyond 4 hours; therefore, it is highly important to eat a mid-afternoon meal or snack, depending on your hunger level. Most women should be eating approximately 1,500 calories per day, and that is the approximate number of calories you'll find in each Skinny Chicks meal plan.

If you don't know exactly how many calories a food contains, don't panic. I tell my clients to eat a protein such as a grilled salmon fillet or chicken breast about the size of their palm. Then I tell them to have a healthy carb such as rice pilaf or a sweet potato about the size of their clenched fist with the other hand wrapped around it. A portion of fat

Skinny Chick Chat

DEAR CHRISTINE: I'm having a difficult time keeping track of every little calorie. I'm trying to stay within my limits, but sometimes the calorie count is just not available to me (if I'm eating out, for instance) or I forget to read the label. Any suggestions?

BONNIE C.

BONNIE: Don't feel like you have to be a slave to the calorie count. If you're not sure about numbers, use the palm/fist measurement. If you feel that you're putting on weight, then you need to add up your nutrition facts. But chances are, if you're eating the foods from the Skinny Chicks meal plans, you'll stay well within your calorie range.

EAT WELL, CHRISTINE

should be approximately the size of a shot glass for nuts and ½ a shot glass for oils. This is a rough estimate. A snack should be about half the size (and calories) of a regular meal.

The Source of Your Calories

In theory, one calorie is just like any other. Remember the old riddle – which is heavier, a pound of bricks or a pound of feathers? It's a trick question, because a pound is a pound is a pound. So, in theory, it shouldn't matter whether you eat carbs, protein or fat, as long as the calories add up to the right number. It shouldn't matter whether you eat 500 calories of chicken or 500 calories of chicken fat. As long as someone eats 500 fewer calories per day, they should lose 1 pound per week according to 'the numbers'. (1 pound = 3,500 calories; 7 days × 500 calories = 3,500 calories.) But we're not purely talking numbers here; we're talking health as well. We're talking nutrition. So we want to set certain parameters for nutritional content that will keep our calories within a healthy, blood sugar-stabilizing range. To achieve this, we should consume a mix of carbohydrates, protein and fat, in these proportions:

- 50 to 60 per cent carbohydrates (approximately the size of 1½ fists)
- 25 to 30 per cent proteins (approximately the size of your palm)
- 15 to 20 per cent fats (approximately the size of a shot glass for nuts or ½ shot glass for oils).

These are not percentages you want to add up at the end of the day; you want this balance at each and every meal. The body is not a cash register. The balance of nutrients you consume at every meal is the most crucial piece of the puzzle, and we will cover it in detail in the next chapter.

CHAPTER 4

The Beauty of Balance

Every trendy diet programme has its 'magic bullet'. The Atkins diet had its 'no carbs' rule, the Sugar Busters diet had no sugar, the cabbage soup diet had . . . well . . . cabbage soup. The Skinny Chicks programme is not a diet; it is a healthy lifestyle nutrition programme. Therefore it offers no magic bullet for weight loss. However, I do have a golden rule of eating, and it's as simple as it is effective: *eat a combo of protein and carbs at every meal.* Why? Because it is the most effective way to stabilize blood sugar levels with food (apart from memorizing the glycaemic index). Follow this straightforward guideline every time you eat, and I promise you that you will see results.

Dispelling the No-Carb Myth

There are three primary energy-yielding nutrients in our food: protein, carbs and fats. These are known as macronutrients. Our bodies can break down these macronutrients into life-sustaining energy that can be used by our cells. But that's not all we need. We also need to consume vitamins and minerals (micronutrients) in order for the body to work; however, we do not obtain energy from micronutrients. Only protein, carbs and fats give our bodies the energy we need to sustain life.

We now know that the carbs in our food are turned into glucose, which is in turn delivered by the insulin FatEx service. Some of that glucose is dumped into your bloodstream and used immediately by your cells for energy; some is converted into glycogen, the form of glucose that is stored in your muscles and liver; whatever is left over goes into storage and is, basically, what makes you fat (or fatter).

Unfortunately, many people reduce the entire study of nutrition down to two words: 'No carbs.' And these people are absolutely right. By cutting out carbs they *will* lose fat – along with their muscle tissue and their sanity.

What happens to a person who adopts the 'no carb' mantra? You get the three-times-per-day cave-ins and the late-night sweet binges. You get overwhelming cravings for cookies you wake up in the middle of the night to eat. The body needs carbs and it doesn't care how it gets them. Sooner or later your body will win and get its carbohydrate fix – usually in an extra-large quantity.

Let's do another review of how our bodies respond to our real lives. Often, when we get on a health kick, we get up in the morning and have a nice, tall glass of ice-cold orange juice for breakfast. What could be healthier? But when you drink the orange juice (a very sugar-rich carbohydrate) on an empty stomach, your blood sugar level rises rapidly and insulin rushes into the bloodstream. You feel energized because there is glucose in your system to feed your brain, but this rapid rise in blood sugar doesn't last. In a couple of hours you feel very hungry and fatigued. You go into a state known as brain fog, which can only be cured by a trained professional at your local coffee shop. If you miss your coffee break, look out! Around 11 a.m., your body rapidly releases adrenaline and you are in a state of near-panic hunger. You feel like a depraved madwoman as you grab a doughnut and cackle, 'I've got you now, my pretty!' Most of us buy into the 'I'm starving, so I must be losing weight' myth, but the truth is just the opposite. If all you've had was orange juice, coffee and a doughnut, you have flooded your system with glucose, and it is possible that even this small breakfast caused some fat storage because you had too many carbs at once.

Suppose that instead of just having a glass of OJ for breakfast, you also have a delicious egg white scramble. With some protein in your system, your blood sugar level elevates more slowly. The presence of protein in a meal causes the body to prolong satiety and keep blood sugar stable longer than with a non-protein meal. You feel energized and alert – basically like a human being again. Furthermore, because you haven't had too much glucose flooding your bloodstream at once, you minimize the amount of excess being stored as fat and you feel satisfied instead of stressed out.

The PC Combo Solution

The simple solution is . . . eating a combination of protein and carbs with every meal. Skinny Chicks don't eat salads, they eat PC Combos!

It seems too simple to make a difference, but when you follow this rule consistently, you'll find that it makes a big difference. As with most successful couples, it's all about chemistry, and a protein/carb combo is a match made in heaven. Your blood sugar is stable when amino acids (proteins) accompany glucose (carbohydrates) while travelling through the bloodstream. The reason? Proteins naturally lower the glycaemic index (rate of sugar release) of a carbohydrate. Thus, combining proteins with carbs helps stabilize blood sugar; prolongs energy and satiety; and makes weight loss so much easier.

If you're wondering where fats fit into all this, truth be told, fats also lower the glycaemic index of a carbohydrate. But, here's my advice: the majority of us don't have to put a lot of thought and effort into making sure we consume the necessary amount of fat. We'll get our 20 per cent with or without trying. Any effort you expend on the fat front should go into making sure you're getting enough 'good' fats; more on that later. What's important to remember is that when it comes to meals or snack time, look for a PC Combo.

Merging Onto the Blood Sugar Freeway

Think about the insulin FatEx van cruising through the bloodstream. I call it the Blood Sugar Freeway (BSF). Ever been in a hurry to get to the

Skinny Chick 10-Week Transformation

NAME: LEZLIE W.

AGE: 25

TOTAL POUNDS LOST: 1 (0.5 kg)

TOTAL INCHES LOST: 1 (2.5 cm)

EMOTION LOST: CHRONIC DEPRESSION

EMOTION GAINED: JOY AND HAPPINESS

(Sometimes it's not just about weight. Lezlie is a model and did not need to lose weight, but she was curious about nutrition and her sessions with me changed the course of her life for ever. Read on.)

I have suffered from anxiety and depression from early childhood. As I reached puberty, the hormones only made it worse. When I was at home, we usually ate pasta or some kind of chicken dish. When I was away from home, my diet consisted of sugar, sugar and more sugar. I was always a skinny girl. All of the other girls were developing curves, and I was still a bean-pole. At the time, I didn't appreciate it, and I remember doing things like eating bowls of ice cream before bed in hopes of putting on some weight.

By the time I started university, I had finally put on some weight and developed the curves I had dreamed about for years, only to find that the attention made me insecure rather than happy. I began a cycle of binge eating.

At the same time, I began to experience extreme mood fluctuations. I remember watching TV with a boyfriend one night: the sound from the bag of crisps he was eating began to drive me mad, so much so that I envisioned throwing him out of the window.

After uni, I decided to pursue the arts full time. The first year was almost enough to send me back home in tears. But somehow, by the grace of God, I made it through.

I turned to prescription drugs to help me gain some control over my depression and anxiety, which regularly caused me to miss auditions and classes. I went from a US size 4 (UK 6), 8 stone 13 pounds (57 kilograms), to a US size 8 (UK 10), and 10 stone 2 pounds (65 kilograms). During the months when I took medication, I felt extremely calm. However, those around me would mention that I wasn't 'me'. Apparently, I became a zombie. I didn't care, though; I'd rather be a zombie than a monster.

And then I began Christine's nutrition programme. On the first day, when Christine listed the symptoms of hypoglycaemia, I looked at her in wonder; could it be that I had been treating hypoglycaemia with depression medication? No one had ever mentioned hypoglycaemia to me before. And when I met with my psychologist, he never asked me about my eating habits, only about my emotional state.

I decided that if I began to feel better on Christine's programme, I would come off the medication. After 3 weeks of her regime, I felt healthier than I ever had in my whole life. My mood was sunny; I had fewer 'nerves'. And, with the help of my doctor, I was able to wean myself off of my medicine. And I hope my story will encourage other women who suffer from depression and anxiety. After trying everything under the sun, it was this programme that really helped me conquer my demons.

airport when the freeway (motorway) is clogged with traffic? I have, and it isn't fun. But when you are on the freeway driving to the airport and there is no traffic, you zip right through in a matter of minutes. This is great if you're in a car. In your body, however, you actually *want* traffic on the Blood Sugar Freeway because when glucose (from carbs) is alone in the bloodstream, it zips right through to fat storage.

Let's go back to that morning glass of OJ for a moment. When you drink the juice, your body releases a fleet of insulin FatEx vans to carry little parcels of this new glucose to its trillions of cells. If your cells' glucose levels are low (which they are if you haven't eaten for more than 5 hours), the FatEx van leaves a parcel of glucose in your cells. Once all the cells are full of energy/glucose, the FatEx van dumps the extra glucose in the body's storage containers: fat cells. When the Blood Sugar Freeway is empty, the FatEx van makes its deliveries so quickly that there is more glucose than your cells need, causing much to be stored as fat.

Now, let's imagine you had that egg white scramble with your orange juice. (And, while we're at it, let's scramble in some green onions, tomatoes and cheese – a radical concept for us girls: a civilized breakfast.) Inside your body, the egg protein is broken down into amino acids that also enter the bloodstream. Now there's some traffic on the Blood Sugar Freeway, and it takes the FatEx van longer to deliver its glucose parcels. Protein is causing your body to release amino acids onto the Blood Sugar Freeway to help stabilize your blood sugar. This added traffic on the BSF helps your body receive glucose energy slowly over a period of hours, keeping your energy steady until lunchtime. When it comes to weight loss, your cells need a steady supply of glucose, not a glucose feast or famine. So even though traffic is the bane of your existence in real life, you actually want your insulin FatEx van to be stuck in slow-moving traffic on the Blood Sugar Freeway.

The Balancing Act

Nutrition is not just about losing fat. It is also about getting all the vitamins and minerals (micronutrients) you need. The greater a variety of healthy foods you eat, the more likely it is that you will get enough vitamins and minerals. For that reason, you need to eat a balance of starchy, high-fibre carbs – wholewheat pasta, brown rice, wholemeal bread – and nutrient-packed carbs – fruits and vegetables. Healthy starchy carbs give you more of the energy you need to survive, and they are packed with fibre (which helps to stabilize blood sugar), vitamins, minerals and antioxidants.

Another reason to eat a balance of protein, carbs and fats at every meal is that it is far more satisfying. When you eat this way, you feel like you're eating real, honest food because, well, you *are*. You have a nice feeling of fullness for a longer time. It's not the same lethargic, bloated feeling of fullness you get from gorging on chocolate cake; it is a healthy, steady energy. Once my clients find out what is going on inside their bodies, they no longer feel so stressed out about their food choices. After 1 week on my programme, a client told me she hadn't felt so relaxed about food and eating for 2 decades.

The Protein/Carb/Fat Formula

Now that you understand how important it is to have a PC Combo at every meal, you're probably wondering how much of the P to combine with the C. As a general rule, to maintain optimum blood sugar levels for weight loss, you should eat roughly two parts carbohydrates to one part protein. As we learned in the previous chapter, you should obtain 25 to 30 per cent of your calories from lean protein sources. Roughly double this amount (50 to 60 per cent) of your calories should come from healthy carbs and the remainder (15 to 20 per cent) should come from healthy fats. (For lists of lean proteins, healthy carbs and good fats, see the Appendix starting on page 275.)

Remember that these are calorie measurements, not volume or weight measurements, so don't go and measure these out on scales. Fats pack a very large number of calories in a very small space compared with carbohydrates or even most proteins. That's why a few pats of butter might have the same number of calories as a whole plate of pasta. The only way to get these calorie balances truly perfect is to read

DIVIDE YOUR PLATE

FRUITS AND VEGETABLES

PROTEIN

STARCHY CARBS

the labels of every food and add up the calories, and although this is tedious, I often advise my clients to do just that, especially when beginning the programme. The good news is that once you get the hang of it, you won't have to pay such meticulous attention to calorie counts and you can use your hand as a guide for portion control. For most people, the right balance looks like this: protein, such as grilled chicken breast, lean steak or fish roughly the size of your palm; a delicious starchy, high-fibre carb such as pasta or rice, roughly the size of your closed fist with your opposite hand wrapped around it; and two scoops of healthy vegetables. You can also think of it this way: divide your plate into four and fill one quarter with protein. Fill another quarter with a starchy carb. The remaining two quarters should be filled with healthy fruits or vegetables (see the Appendix). Use a small amount (no more than a tablespoon) of healthy fats such as olive oil for cooking or additional flavour.

If you are still not sure how much you should be eating, check out the meal plans starting on page 122; they'll give you a lot of great meal ideas that don't require you to weigh or measure every item.

But beware of sticking to the letter of this healthy habit while ignoring the spirit behind it. For instance, I once had a client who loved jelly beans; she would literally eat a grilled chicken breast with a handful of these little sweets. Was she successful at losing weight? As a matter of fact, she was. But she was feeding her body a food that had absolutely no nutritional value whatsoever. Depriving your body of the nutrients it needs deprives you of living your best, healthiest life. Plus, if you don't nurture your body along the way, sooner or later you'll come up against a mountain of health problems. Eating a healthy balance means eating not only a PC Combo but also a variety of foods to get all the vitamins and minerals your body needs. If I were to help you succeed in losing weight but let you become sick due to vitamin deficiencies, I wouldn't be much of a nutritionist. So be adventurous and eat a wide variety of healthy foods.

CHAPTER 5

Munch around the Clock

One, two, three o'clock, four o'clock munch.
Five, six, seven o'clock, eight o'clock crunch.
Nine, ten, eleven o'clock, twelve o'clock lunch.
We're gonna munch around the clock today!

In 1953, Bill Haley and the Comets had a revolutionary idea that went against what most people thought of as 'the norm'. Haley wanted everyone to rock around the clock. Well, now it's time for another revolutionary rockin' idea: munch around the clock.

If you're eating to stabilize your blood sugar levels so that you can lose weight and live your healthiest life, *when* you eat is just as important as *what* you eat. When it comes to losing weight, most people try to eat less often, and less food at each meal, thinking food deprivation is the ticket to weight loss. They couldn't be more wrong! This chapter will help ease that confusion.

Here's what you need to know: Skinny Chicks eat every 4 hours, whether it's a complete meal or a snack. This will keep your blood sugar at a consistent level. This doesn't mean have breakfast at 7 a.m. and lunch at 12 p.m.; it means if you eat your first meal at 7 a.m., have lunch at 11 a.m. Then have another lunch or a snack at 3 p.m. and eat dinner at 7 p.m. If you eat at 7.30 p.m. and you are up until 12 midnight, you should eat a PC Combo meal before bed. My clients do this all the time and still continue to lose weight. Of course if you are not that hungry, I recommend you eat a smaller meal . . . but you need to eat *something*. Of course I realize this is contrary to what people normally do in order to lose weight. However, on the Skinny Chicks programme you *need* to eat every 4 hours in order to avoid those sugar binges.

If you eat only when you are ravenously hungry, you will have waited until your body is out of stored glucose. Your blood sugar level will be down in the basement and you'll feel it. You'll lose your ability to concentrate, you'll feel lightheaded and you'll probably experience physical hunger 'pangs'. And you know what happens then – you start to hear that voice in your head that says, 'Eat! Eat!' And it's not saying, 'Eat a big piece of fish'. Your brain needs fuel and will work hard to convince you to go and get the most carbohydrate-laden snack you can find.

Starving yourself sets you up to crave all the foods you *shouldn't* be eating. If, instead, you have a PC Combo every 4 hours, your blood sugar will love you for it and you'll set yourself up to choose the right foods.

The Clock Strikes 'Carb'

Blood sugar levels drop dramatically 3 to 4 hours after a meal, regardless of the amount of carbohydrates previously consumed. If you had an overabundance of carbohydrates in your previous meal, just remember that the FatEx van is busy driving around, delivering special parcels in various places on your body, giving you more lumps, bumps, hips and thighs than your body wants or needs.

It's when we are too busy to eat that we get into trouble. We get too involved in what we are doing, and we think we'll save time by hitting the vending machine. We tell ourselves, 'I'm starving and I don't have time for a real meal, so I'll just have a handful of crisps.' What happens then?

A handful turns into half the bag, and half the bag becomes the whole lot, and sometimes even that's not enough. Not long after, you notice that all the salt from the crisps has made you extremely thirsty, so you reach for a large fizzy drink. Why? First, when salt is absorbed into the bloodstream, it makes the fluid outside your cells saltier than the fluid inside your cells. That extra salt essentially calls out to the salt inside the cells and says, 'Hey, come on out here and play'. The cell, always the goody two-shoes and looking for balance, e-mails the brain and says, 'There's too much salt floating around outside. Send me some help.' That's when you start to feel thirsty. All that extra salt also increases the amount of electrolytes in our blood. Electrolytes carry the electrical impulses that help control our bodily functions. Too many electrolytes turns on the thirst centre, and we need liquids to get us back in balance again. That's why, when you go into a bar, you'll often find peanuts free for the taking. Those clever bar owners know that those salty snacks will have us ordering more drinks quicker than Shakira can shake her booty.

And that's also why we reach for something sweet to drink. We all know that sweet flavours taste phenomenal with salty flavours. So you gulp down a fizzy drink, and 750 calories later, you feel energized, yet puffy and borderline depressed.

It is far better to stop what you are doing for 5 minutes and prepare yourself a PC Combo, like a turkey sandwich or a bowl of fruit with cottage cheese. If you make this part of your daily routine, you won't get to the point where your body is craving the crisps and chocolates. You won't even miss them at all!

Why You Need to Eat Every 4 Hours

Imagine this scenario: you're a contestant on *Survivor: Skinny Chicks Island*. You haven't eaten anything but a few ugly bugs for 24 hours. Suddenly, you come across a wild bird sitting on a nest of six eggs. You quickly scoop them up and hide them in your pockets. You are tempted to eat all six at once, but your instincts tell you otherwise, so you eat one now and save the rest for later, one every few hours. That way you will spread out your energy resources as long as possible.

That's an extreme example, but you get the idea. If you ate all the eggs at once, you'd have consumed extra calories your body would not be able to use that would just go to waste (or to waist, as the case may be). This is essentially what happens when you eat three large meals a day with many hours in between each meal. By eating smaller meals every 4 hours, your body gets just the right amount of energy and uses it for the fuel it needs.

Many studies have shown that eating smaller, more frequent meals is not only better for losing weight, but better for your general health as well. One early study, published in 1989, divided participants into two separate groups. Both groups were given the same number of calories to consume each day, but one group ate a regular breakfast, lunch and dinner while the second group was fed 17 small snacks throughout the day. At the end of the study, the 'nibblers' had lowered their cholesterol by 14 per cent and decreased their average insulin level by 28 per cent.

Another study, from the US *Proceedings of the National Academy of Sciences*, suggested that if you want to keep thinking, you've got to keep eating. Have you ever noticed that your ability to concentrate decreases as your hunger increases? You're not imagining things. The study found that ' . . . cognitive ability can deplete extra-cellular glucose in the hippocampus . . . ', the region of the brain critical for learning and memory, and that ' . . . exogenous glucose administration reverses the depletion while enhancing task performance'. In other words, thinking is hard work that causes the brain to use up energy supplies faster than do other regions of the body during critical problem solving. The only way to get your cognitive abilities up to par once again is to feed the brain more glucose by having a snack or a meal. Obviously, the best way to keep your brain train on track at all times is to keep it continuously supplied with fuel *before it becomes depleted*, which means eating every 4 hours.

Here are some other reasons to munch around the clock:

- Muscle tissue is better preserved when you eat every 4 hours. This is good because more muscle means a faster metabolism.

- Liver tissue is preserved if you eat every 4 hours. This is good because a healthy liver also means a faster metabolism.

Skinny Chick Chat

DEAR CHRISTINE: What happens when fat stores are used up? Where do those fat cells go?

JOANNE C.

JOANNE: Actually, except for a small percentage of fat cells, they don't go anywhere. A new study reported in the *New York Times* found that every year, no matter how fat or thin you are, or whether you lose or put on weight, 10 per cent of your fat cells die. However, every year the cells that die are replaced by new fat cells. The result is that the number of fat cells in your body remains the same throughout your adult life. Losing weight only affects the amount of fat stored in the cells, not the number of cells, and the same goes for gaining weight. Overweight people have more fat cells in their bodies than thin people do. Even people who have had weight loss surgery and lost a significant amount of weight possess the same number of fat cells they had before the surgery — even if they have become much thinner. One theory, called the fat cell hypothesis, says that the number of fat cells is determined early in life, and after that they can change only in size, not in number. When people lose weight and the fat cells shrink, the cells send hormonal signals asking to be filled up again. That's why most people regain weight that they have lost. Unfortunately, scientists are still searching for ways to turn off that signal. In the mean time, the best way to get those fat cells to shrink and 'stay shrunk' is to follow the Skinny Chicks programme.

EAT WELL, CHRISTINE

- The brain needs a constant, steady stream of glucose for survival. Brain cells use up to twice as much blood sugar as any other cell in the body.

- It's nice to eat often. Who doesn't like to eat?

Running on Empty

When a car runs out of petrol and conks out, it just stops moving. There is no reserve tank it can switch to for more fuel. Remember that when we humans run out of petrol (blood sugar – Tank 1), we don't conk out because we do have reserve tanks: glycogen in liver and muscle tissue (Tank 2), our lean tissues and organs (Tank 3) and body fat (ketosis – Tank 4). The body doesn't conk out like a car because it starts eating through its own engine. If you are running on nothing but caffeine all day, you are borrowing energy from your own body. But that's good, isn't it? Don't we want to burn our own body fat for energy?

Unfortunately, the body doesn't work that simply. This is why there are so many overweight people and also why so much money is poured into the industry of weight-loss advice. After glucose from food runs out, your body accesses some body fat, but it goes after glycogen stored in your liver tissue first. Then, after a few more hours, your body begins to convert muscle tissue to glucose (a process called glycogenolysis, the biochemical breakdown of glycogen to glucose). Now your metabolism slows to a crawl and fat burning in your body is minimized. Furthermore, you are starving and you feel miserable and cranky. Only after about 24 to 72 hours (depending on the individual) does your body begin to significantly access body fat for energy. But as we observed in Chapter 3, there are very few of us who can actually hold out for a full 3 days without eating (or simply without eating carbs). If you are strong-willed enough to get through the 72 hours of carb deprivation, you will lose weight. But before you go on a hunger strike, remember this: your metabolic rate will also be slower because your muscle and liver tissues will have been compromised. Worst of all, you will put back on most if not all of the weight once you begin to eat 'real' food again.

Skinny Chick 10-Week Transformation

NAME: RAHA T.

AGE: 20

TOTAL POUNDS LOST: 16 (7.3 kg)

TOTAL INCHES LOST: 22.5 (57 cm)

When I was young, I was really, really thin – so thin that my ribs stuck out. Then puberty came along and so did a tyre around my waist. I was the only girl around with big boobs and a big stomach. I always felt like the biggest girl in the room.

I was a compulsive dieter, but nothing really worked. I suffered from depression and anxiety, and that made me lose weight, but 5 minutes later I would put it back on again. I was stuck in a compulsive dieting/eating cycle.

What I learned from Christine's programme is that starvation doesn't work, and it's OK to have carbs. You need carbs to sustain your life. And I learned that you need to combine protein and carbs, so I can have chicken and rice for dinner, which I love, and it's been working.

This programme has actually created a lot of balance in my life because of the scheduling. I'm now eating really good food every 4 hours. When the 4 hours are up, I can't wait to eat my yogurt and fruit, or whatever I'm having. My life is now scheduled around these 4-hour intervals, and it works perfectly. When I went shopping and bought my first batch of food, it all fell into place for me and it was really easy from then on!

By week 3, I was already looking different and people were asking if I had lost weight. I slept really well at night and found I woke up even before my alarm went off. I don't have cravings any more. And not only that – people have seen a significant difference in my attitude. I'm not as moody. I've never been so happy.

Several days without adequate food would mean a tremendous metabolic slowdown. The fat inside each fat cell cannot get out and actually leave your body in a healthy and permanent way unless you can keep the Blood Sugar Freeway moving. It wants out but everything has come to a screeching halt, because if you do not eat frequent meals, your body will hold on to stored fat and slow down cellular processes in an effort to conserve fuel/energy.

Midnight Munchies

Now, I'm not going to ask you to get up in the middle of the night to continue the every-4-hours pattern. You don't need as much energy while you're sleeping, and your body will dip into its reserve fuel sources to get what it does need. But you must eat breakfast within 1 hour of waking. And if you eat every 4 hours during the day, your blood sugar will be stabilized throughout the day and your hormones will be more balanced, which aids sleep. Furthermore, sleeping for 8 hours actually helps your body keep weight off, so you should spend your nights in dreamland instead of foodland. The good news is that you won't be hungry at night because you have eaten solid, fulfilling PC Combo meals throughout the day and into the evening.

CHAPTER 6

Every Body's Got Issues

Okay. Here's another quick quiz, and this one's a breeze.

- Quick – without thinking about it, name five parts of your body you truly love.
- Now, without thinking about it, name five parts of your body you can't stand.

Which one of those lists was easier to make? I can almost guarantee it was the second one, and I wouldn't be surprised if you came up with more than five. It's a sad fact of the world we live in today that we judge ourselves and our imperfections so harshly. Even the skinniest of chicks has areas that make her unhappy. We are embarrassed to be in our own skins.

Through my experience with thousands of clients, I've learned that people cannot lose weight successfully if they are in the midst of an internal battle. One of two things will happen:

1. They will lose the weight out of self-hate and disgust, which often becomes an eating disorder, or

2. When they do make progress and lose weight, they will allow negative thoughts to steal their joy and tell them that they really have not progressed, which brings self-defeat and sends them into a binge eating frenzy.

You Are What You Think

Many health gurus say 'you are what you eat', which is somewhat true; however, my mantra is 'you are what you think'. A large portion of my nutrition consulting appointments are spent explaining to my clients that they must change their thoughts about themselves before they can succeed with weight loss. If they think of themselves as fit and healthy, it will become reality.

I can tell you that on this programme you will lose weight and have more energy within the first week. I can also tell you that if you continue to let negative thoughts about your body into your mind, you will have a very difficult time losing weight. I've seen these thoughts drive away my clients' hopes of ever improving their shape and health. It's as if the body senses your view of yourself and makes it reality by not allowing the weight to come off. After years of dealing with both people who are overweight and those who are in wonderful shape, I've learned that our thoughts and words hold the power to keep us where we are or get us where we want to go. So, before you begin my weight loss programme, I would like you to make an effort to release all the negative thoughts you have about your body and begin to use healthy thoughts and healthy words in your life. You need healthy thoughts to inspire healthy actions.

I know all about body issues. I was a catwalk model at 12, a swimsuit model in my teens and in my early twenties, I appeared on the cover of fitness magazines. To be a successful fitness model, you have to be lean, cut, chiselled – flawless. You can't go to a photo shoot with your stomach protruding even a tiny bit, so you don't eat breakfast. You don't eat lunch. By 3 in the afternoon, you're ready to faint – but you don't dare eat. You're standing there as a representation of perfect health while you're actually dying inside because your body is breaking down muscle

Skinny Chick Chat

DEAR CHRISTINE: I've been following the Skinny Chicks programme for several weeks now and making progress. But my friend Sheila, who's also on the programme, is losing weight faster than I am. Last week, she lost 4 pounds (1.8 kilograms) and I only lost a pound and a half (685 grams). What am I doing wrong?

JANINE F.

HERE'S MY ADVICE TO YOU, JANINE: Stay in your own lane. Don't look at the person next to you to see how well you're doing. Your weight loss is fantastic! In the first few weeks of the Skinny Chicks test group, several of the women were constantly comparing themselves with others in the group. One woman, who had lost 2 pounds (900 grams) that week, went to the back of the room and cried when she saw that another woman had lost 5 pounds (2¼ kilograms). I explained to her that everyone is different and that she shouldn't be disappointed in herself or think that she hadn't done the programme correctly. Even if you don't lose any weight in a particular week, the simple fact that you're no longer going to a fast-food restaurant for lunch or having a bag of crisps for dinner is something to celebrate. Keep track of your own progress, and allow yourself to feel good about it. You worked hard for that weight loss! Enjoy your accomplishment.

EAT WELL, CHRISTINE

and liver tissue in order to survive. You do whatever you need to do to keep that perfect body perfect. And all the while, you think you're fat.

When I was 5 feet 9 inches (1.75 metres) and 8 stone 6 pounds (53.5 kilograms), I struggled with negative body image. I thought I was defective and deformed. Imagine how I felt when I weighed 11 stone 1 lb (70.3 kilograms), and everything in between. I knew I was unhealthy and I never felt good about myself. But the moment I learned the ABCs of nutrition, all of my negative body image thoughts went away. Once I understood how to eat for health, I somehow found peace and calm. Knowing how food and our hormones work internally gave me self-assurance that I was on my way. And it was at that moment that the body image issues went away for ever. It was truly a miracle from God. I weighed over 11 stone (70 kilograms), and, for the first time in my life, I loved myself and my body just as it was. I knew I had a way to go to reach my desired weight, but I found peace in knowing how to get there healthily. I didn't care how long it took; I was just happy to be at peace in my own skin. I hope and pray that this book will offer the same peace to you.

Balance, Blood Sugar and Body Image

How was I able to turn my attitude around? By calling a truce between my mind and my body. When I was eating just ice cream, or subsisting on salads during the day and binge foods at night, my blood sugar was so out of whack that it was literally driving me crazy. Once I began to understand the concept of the PC Combo and eat healthy foods, I could think clearly. The moodiness and depression began to recede, allowing me to develop a more realistic and accepting perspective on my own body.

Being out of balance causes the vicious cycle that makes you overeat and then hate yourself and then eat more and then hate yourself even more and then starve yourself and start all over again. When you learn to stabilize your blood sugar, you eliminate the cravings and the madness that precipitate all the negative self-talk. You can learn to love the body you have and, if you so choose, find the 'skinny' that's best for you in a smart, healthy way. If you love your life and love your body, you will want to take care of it. We all know how much effort it takes to eat a healthy meal or to get yourself to the gym when everything seems hopeless. However, if you follow the Skinny Chicks programme, balanced meals and moderate exercise will become a fundamental part of your overall lifestyle philosophy, and you will begin almost immediately to feel better about yourself. Instead of seeing yourself in a negative light, you will develop a fundamental identification with health and a love of life, just as I have.

Skinny Chick 10-Week Transformation

NAME: MELIDA N.

AGE: 20

TOTAL POUNDS LOST: 11 (5 kg)

TOTAL INCHES LOST: 20½ (52 cm)

Growing up, I was never really fat – I've always been the 'chubby' one. But I never felt like I fitted in, especially because I was brought up in Germany, where everyone was tall, skinny and blonde. I was constantly teased at school.

My mother was very conscious of my weight. She had always been thin, and she made a point of telling me that I was not. She started putting me on diets when I was 9, and she signed me up for every sport she could find. When you are 9 and your mum is telling you in an indirect way that you're not good enough, it affects your body image. You feel that your mother is disappointed or is ashamed of you. By the time I was 12, I had an eating disorder. It began when my mum put me on a diet where you had to drink vinegar before every meal. I would take some before breakfast, and by the time I got to school, I had to throw up. My mother thought the diet was really working. She was happy because I was losing weight, not realizing what I was doing. Then I found out that a cousin was doing the same thing, so I thought, 'It must be OK because other people are doing it too.'

I came to the United States in 2000, where I literally got introduced to a different world. Here, people are more accepting of who you are – different shapes and sizes and different cultures. And my cousins here weren't all super skinny. I started to realize that even if I was gaining my mum's acceptance, it really wasn't good for me. I was tired all the time. I was becoming ill more often.

Christine's programme helped me get over my eating disorder and bad eating habits by showing me that I can eat every 4 hours and have great food that I love, and still lose weight and be healthy. She showed me that I don't have to hate food. Food is not my enemy. I can love food and be healthy.

Christine stresses to listen to your body. Often I haven't been doing this. I wasn't good to my body when it was telling me not to starve myself. I think that phrase is really important: *love your body, listen to your body*. It's inspiring because you see results. When people give you compliments, it boosts your self-esteem. That's really important in how you carry yourself and how you look at life. Because of this programme, I'm thinking things like *I can go to medical school, I can lose weight, I can live a better life*. It's really exciting.

Stop Comparing and Start Dreaming Big

Body image issues are exacerbated when we compare ourselves with others, whether it's friends and family, actresses or models. There is no one who compares to you. There will always be people who are thinner, or richer or more successful than you – at this time. Tomorrow, you may be at the top of the heap. Either way, what matters is that you believe in yourself and your self-worth no matter what anyone else has, does or achieves.

Adopt a mind-set that says 'I'm a Skinny Chick' even if you're not. If you have a mind-set that says 'I'm always going to be overweight and unattractive and I'm never going to be anything different', guess what? That's what you're going to get. If it's not in your heart, it's not really going to make a difference in your life. You have to believe it.

PART II

SKINNY CHICKS

REVISIT PROTEIN

AND CARBS

CHAPTER 7

Lean, Mean Protein

Growing up, I remember Sunday lunches at my grandparents' farm in California. By noon, the house was filled with smells of a traditional Italian family dinner: fresh, homemade Italian pasta with a savoury red meat sauce. My grandmother used meats of every sort in her sauce: chicken, turkey, beef, pork or even fish and seafood. The smell of the meat – sautéeing in the onions, garlic and spices – wafted throughout the house and drifted outside, where I was playing with my cousins. Before long, my large extended family would be lining up at the table. The meal was delicious and incredibly satisfying to all of us kids after playing outside all day.

It never occurred to me to wonder whether it was a healthy meal, or how I could eat and eat my grandmother's pasta and never put on any weight, even as I got older.

Eventually, I moved to San José in pursuit of the excitement of the big city and forgot all about the simplicity of youth. Somewhere in the 1980s and 1990s, pasta became a forbidden treat and Italian food was seen as old-fashioned and passé. Pizza, pasta with Parmesan, even good old spaghetti were considered health *faux pas*. For a short while in the mid 1990s, the accepted wisdom in health and nutrition circles was to cut out pasta entirely.

Maybe that's why – get ready for a big revelation – I cook a huge pasta dinner for myself and my husband and any guests we might have every Sunday night. While I'm sautéeing the meat, the incredible, savoury aromas of onions, garlic, hot chilli peppers and extra virgin olive oil fill the whole house. I always add chicken, prawns, salmon or turkey mince. Whichever I choose, the primary element is the protein, and the most important part of the preparation is browning the meat. If you just add spice to meat after it is cooked, it will wash off in the sauce and end up tasting bland. However, if you sautée your meat with spices, the meat will burst with flavour in your mouth and it will make all the difference.

So, on Sunday nights we eat pasta to our heart's content, and yes, Mick Jagger, you *can* get satisfaction, because this dinner is fulfilling and satisfying. And it's not because of the pasta or the tomatoes; it's because of the protein. And that's the subject of this chapter: protein.

Almost everything we think of when we think of our bodies is made from protein: our cells, tissues and organs; our hair, skin, blood, bones and muscles. Protein is one of the three nutrients (along with fats and carbs) that provide calories to the body – 4 calories per gram, in fact. At the end of this chapter, you'll find a list of the healthiest sources of protein for the Skinny Chicks programme.

Here's what protein does for your metabolism:

- It helps stabilize blood sugar, enabling you to burn more fat between meals.

- It keeps you feeling fuller longer and minimizes the munchies.

- It slows the absorption and digestion of sugars (carbohydrates) and can lower the glycaemic index of high glycaemic index carbs (more on the glycaemic index in Chapter 8).

- It helps maintain muscle mass, which keeps metabolism humming.

The Real Skinny on Protein and Belly Fat

Researchers at the Royal Veterinary and Agricultural University in Copenhagen found that women and men who consumed at least 25 per cent of their daily calories as protein lost 10 per cent more belly fat than those who consumed just 12 per cent of their calories as protein. This is important news, because belly fat is a danger sign of poor health. It turns out this kind of fat (called visceral fat) releases harmful hormones, turns into cholesterol in the bloodstream (which eventually turns into artery-clogging plaque), secretes substances that cause inflammation and decreases the body's sensitivity to insulin. Although researchers are not exactly sure why eating more protein reduces belly fat, one theory says that it's possible that protein intake may trigger smaller releases of the stress hormone cortisol, which directs the body to store fat in the tummy area. Less cortisol, less muffin top!

By now, you know that the mainstay of the Skinny Chicks programme is the PC Combo. But do you know why we need to include protein in every meal and snack? Because in order to deliver the benefits above, your body needs a constant supply. And while we can store fats and carbs for future use, we can't store protein. There's no reserve storage facility in the body to replenish the supply, so we have to keep a steady stream coming.

That doesn't mean you should be eating huge amounts of protein every day. We know that adults need a minimum of 0.8 gram of protein per day for every kilogram of body weight (1 kilogram = 2¼ pounds) just to keep from slowly breaking down their own tissues, although I recommend a little more than this. Remember that a serving size of protein is about the size of your palm. In fact, a few grams of protein go a long way, so there's no need to overdo.

More Benefits of Protein

For a woman, protein is the thing that you want the most for the things most important to you: your skin and your hair. There is not a woman (or a man, for that matter) who doesn't want healthy skin and hair. Your skin and hair (along with your muscles, the haemoglobin in your blood, and many enzymes that keep you alive) are made up mostly of protein. Your body takes the proteins you eat, breaks them down into amino acids (the building blocks of proteins), recombines them into new proteins, and makes new skin cells and promotes hair growth. They also create antibodies that fight off infection and disease. If you deprive yourself of protein for a long time, you can say goodbye to healthy skin and hair because there will be no new building blocks for generating new hair and skin cells.

PROTEIN AND WEIGHT LOSS

From a weight-loss standpoint, there are many benefits to protein:

- The most important benefit is that protein creates a hormonal response that triggers fat burning.

- Protein eaten together with carbohydrates will slow the absorption of glucose (sugar from carbs) into the bloodstream, which will keep blood sugar levels more stable and provide steady healthy energy.

- A meal is always much more satisfying when it includes a lean portion of chicken, turkey, fish or beef. And there are plenty of great vegetarian protein sources, too, such as low-fat soya foods like tofu and tempeh, low-fat yogurts and cheeses, and beans or pulses – especially lentils (for a more complete list of vegetarian proteins, see page 277). When you feel sated, you are less inclined to snack between meals.

- When prepared correctly, meats are delicious, which is perhaps the most important thing of all, since you should love what you eat.

How does protein affect fat burning? Protein-rich meals trigger the release of the hormone glucagon, the antagonist hormone of insulin. As you know by now, insulin is a 'storing' (anabolic) hormone. On the other hand, glucagon is a 'mobilizing' (catabolic) hormone. Insulin clears away glucose and packs it away into cells for storage. Glucagon's job is to release glucose from cells when blood sugar levels are too low. According to Dr Balint Kacsoh, author of *Endocrine Physiology*, glucagon also stimulates lipolysis (the breakdown of fat for energy) in adipose tissue (fat) by activating hormone-sensitive lipase. In other words, glucagon is part of a process that ultimately helps break down triglycerides, which are stored body fats, into their component parts: free fatty acids and glycerol. Once these parts are separated, they can leave the fat cell and be used by the body for energy. This effect is subtle yet important, so please do not use this as a green light to load up on protein – remember, healthy weight loss is about eating PC Combos and not protein alone.

Which Proteins to Choose

The short answer is chicken, turkey, fish, egg whites and low-fat dairy products. I eat one of these in nearly every meal, and there are lots of delicious ways to prepare each of them. (See the recipes starting on page 237.) If you are vegetarian or vegan, there are plenty of great choices for you as well (see page 277). If you want to lose weight, you want the leanest proteins, which are those listed above. Then you want to prepare them in a way that doesn't turn them into an oil sponge.

I recommend eating beef no more than once a week due to its high saturated fat content. The leanest cuts are those that include the word 'loin', such as tenderloin or sirloin. If you enjoy steak, I say go ahead and throw a nice sirloin under the grill once a week. Pork is another lean meat for which it's best to choose the 'loin' cuts for pork that is organically raised. Here are some other popular protein choices:

- **Chicken and turkey:** Most of my clients eat a large amount of chicken and turkey. You can buy great-tasting turkey burgers, and you can replace beef mince with turkey mince in most recipes – often, the result is even tastier than the original. Burgers, pasta with meat sauce or meatballs, meat loaf, tacos, and even lasagne and enchiladas can all be made with turkey. Chicken can be sautéed in garlic, onions and spices to provide the flavour base for dozens of great pasta and rice dishes that will not only fill you up but also taste so good they'll knock your socks off. And of course, if you are not inclined towards the kitchen, you can always throw chicken on the grill or buy a ready-roasted chicken.

- **Fish:** Fish is a very lean source of protein. Favourites include salmon, halibut, trout, mackerel and haddock, scallops and prawns. Sushi with salmon, eel, crab and prawns are healthy choices as well as delicious. Tuna is a great protein source, although it is becoming increasingly overfished and endangered. Avoid the scarce bluefin and yellowfin tuna and look for skipjack. I also recommend moderation due to the possibility (albeit small) of trace mercury content. I tell my clients to limit tuna to one 3-ounce (90-gram) serving per week. (The UK Food Standards Agency says it is safe for pregnant women to consume two servings of light tuna per week, but I often advise women who are pregnant or planning on becoming pregnant to avoid all tuna until after they finish breastfeeding.) For further information go to http://www.food.gov.uk/multimedia/faq/mercuryfish/.

- **Eggs:** Eggs are a great source of protein, and there is nothing more satisfying and long-lasting than a hot breakfast with eggs. I always use egg whites with just a little yolk, as the yolks are high in cholesterol and fat. One egg yolk has approximately 4 grams of fat, so it's not the best choice for people who want to lose weight, but egg whites are a great lean source of protein, yielding 3 grams per white.

- **Dairy products:** Dairy products can be deceptive because they offer proteins, carbs and fats in one bite, and they can vary in their protein content. It can present a bit of a challenge for meal preparation. The chart shows that not all yogurt is created equal:

TYPE OF YOGURT	CALORIES PER 170-G (6-OZ) SERVING	PROTEIN (G)	CARBS (G)	FAT (G)	GOOD/BAD PROTEIN SOURCE?
Plain low-fat	75	11	16	2	Good source of protein
Greek, plain low-fat	110	15	7	3	Good source of protein
Plain, whole milk	130	8	11	6	Bad protein source – too much fat
Flavoured, low-fat	157	7	30	1.5	Bad protein source – too many carbs
Flavoured, whole milk	172	8	23	5	Bad protein source – you need 3 servings to get enough protein, thus too many carbs and too much fat
Greek, flavoured, whole milk	283	9	32	14	Bad protein source – too much fat and carbs
Greek, plain, whole milk	221	12	5	17	Bad protein source – too much fat

*Comments based on recommended nutrition parameter of 1 part protein, 2 parts carbohydrates.

Magazine Article Diets

In virtually any magazine in the newsagent, you will find an article offering a quick slim-down diet from doctors known and unknown, fitness trainers, nutritionists, health experts, writers and every other possible person under the sun with a computer. They inevitably recommend the following diet: cereal with milk for breakfast, bagel with peanut butter for a snack, chicken salad for lunch, a handful of nuts for a snack, and a dinner of fish and vegetables. They add up the total protein, carbs and fats for the day and presto: they suggest this is a balanced diet. But

Skinny Chick Chat

DEAR CHRISTINE: I heard that I should stay away from fish because of the possibility of mercury. Can you tell me which types of fish are safe?

TAMIKA

TAMIKA: Your concerns about mercury are valid, but don't throw the baby out with the bathwater. The benefits of fish far outweigh the risks for most individuals. For children and for women who are of childbearing age, or who are pregnant or breast-feeding, mercury is definitely a concern. Mercury, which comes from industrial emissions, burning coal and natural sources, can harm a developing brain and nervous system. Fish that are high in mercury include shark, sword-fish and marlin. Another fish to avoid if you are of childbearing age is albacore tuna, which contains more mercury than light tuna does. (Tinned tuna is the most widely consumed fish.) Stick to light tuna and limit yourself to one serving per week. It is, however, important for everyone to consume at least two portions of fish per week (including one of oily fish) according to the UK Food Standards Agency, so you should still enjoy a variety of wild-caught fresh fish and shellfish. Some of the best are Icelandic cod, halibut, pollock, salmon, sole and trout. (Getting enough omega-3 fatty acids – of which fish are an excellent source – also aids a baby's nervous system development. Be sure to ask your doctor for the latest recommendations on fish consumption.)

For more information on mercury in fish, go to http://www.food.gov.uk/multimedia/faq/mercuryfish.

EAT WELL, CHRISTINE

your body doesn't add things up at the end of the day. It digests the food that's in your stomach at any given moment. I cringe whenever I see all these lightweight meals and snacks. For instance, a bowl of cereal with milk contains a small amount of protein (in the milk), but it's mostly refined carbs. It is neither satisfying nor a truly balanced meal, as there simply is not enough protein. The same goes for a bagel and peanut butter – you are getting a bunch of refined carbs and twice as much fat as protein.

A meal like that might stabilize blood sugar because there is fat and protein in peanut butter, but it won't satisfy your hunger. You feel like you are starving, because you are. Invariably you end up eating a huge dinner to compensate for the day-long deprivation – a dinner with second helpings, two glasses of wine and dessert. Remember that weight gain happens when you take in too much at once and overwhelm the body with too many calories. The whole day of deprivation might cause a small amount of fat burning, but the big dinner will more than make up for it in fat storage. You may not have a massive binge the first night, but give it a few days and it is sure to happen.

The Real Skinny on Bagels for Breakfast

A study from the Rochester Center for Obesity Research in Michigan monitored 30 women who started their day with eggs and toast. The women felt so full and satisfied that they ate 274 fewer calories over the rest of the day than those who had bagels and cream cheese for breakfast.

The best thing to do is spread the calories from the big dinner into the other three meals of the day. Remember the ABCs – especially your 'Cs', because eating every 4 hours is extremely important if you seriously want to lose weight and keep it off. Make every meal you have a balanced meal that includes a healthy protein.

What If You Don't Eat Meat?

Plenty of people do not eat any animal proteins for reasons of personal preference or ethics. Your body doesn't take politics into account, though – it just reacts to the nutrients it receives. Proteins are a tremendously important part of everyone's diet, including vegetarians'. Fortunately, plant-based proteins such as tempeh, tofu, edamame, lentils, split peas and kidney beans can provide many of the benefits you need without ever harming an animal.

My message to vegetarians is the same one I give all my clients: combine a protein with a carb at every meal. You might be thinking to yourself, 'Well, beans are a carbohydrate *and* a protein, so is it OK for me to consider foods such as lentils a prefab carbohydrate-protein combo?' My answer is yes; however, vegetable protein sources are often higher in calories and even fat, so invest some time in learning their nutritional values.

Vegans, unlike vegetarians, eat no meat, eggs or dairy. However, it is really difficult to satisfy your body's nutritional needs from veggie proteins alone, because many of the sources of plant proteins such as soya-beans, nuts and beans and pulses are nutritionally lacking in one way or another. There are many benefits to eating soya, but recent research compiled by the Harvard School of Public Health finds that the benefits might be counterbalanced by the potential risks of consuming too *much*. One study uncovered a possible link to increased risk for certain cancers. Harvard recommends soya in moderation with an upper limit of four servings per week.

Of all the plant-based proteins, beans and pulses are the best because they are a complete protein and there are no known adverse effects from eating them every day. They include beans (e.g., chickpea, butter (lima), broad (fava), haricot (navy), kidney and pinto), peas (e.g. split, yellow and green), and lentils. In places like India, where many people are vegetarians, beans and pulses are a staple food.

In my practice in Los Angeles, I've worked with many vegans. One basically vegan client by the name of Nichole signed up for my 'Fit and Lean Vegetarian' programme and had tremendous success. Here is Nichole's story as taken from her original files:

Nichole H.

Starting: 11 stone 1 lb (70.3 kg), 22% body fat, US size 12 (UK size 14), 2 stone 4 lb (15.5 kg) fat, 9 stone 4 lb (58.9 kg) muscle

Ending: 10 stone 3 lb (64.8 kg), 15% body fat, US size 5 (UK size 8), 1 stone 8½ lb fat (10.2 kg), 9 stone 3½ lb (58.7 kg) muscle

The impressive thing to notice here is that she lost 12 pounds (5.4 kilograms) of body fat and zero pounds of muscle on this programme and she dropped seven sizes! That should tell you that the numbers on the scales are not always the best indicator of a fit and lean person. On page 76 is an example of Nichole's vegetarian diet before she began working with me.

Food Log for Wednesday, 29 March, 2006

(This is before she started the programme.)

TIME OF MEAL	NICHOLE'S FOOD/ FEELING	CALORIES	CHRISTINE'S COMMENTS
7.30 a.m.	Breakfast bar ... *still hungry*	150	Not enough protein or calories; this spikes blood sugar.
8 a.m.	Soya vanilla latte ... *feeling OK*	160	Another high-sugar, low protein food; this spikes blood sugar.
10 a.m.	Apple ... *starving*	120	Again, more carbs, some fibre, no protein; this will keep you hungry.
12.40 p.m.	4 gummy gators ... *starving but hoping that sugar will pick me up*	35	Another blood sugar spike; this will keep you hungry.
1.15 p.m.	Sandwich made with wheat vegan bread, veggie meat (2 slices) and provolone cheese; lettuce, tomato and honey mustard dressing; fake chicken meat pasta salad	680	This looks OK, but fake chicken salad probably has too much fat.
2 p.m.	Two pieces of hard candy	45	Blood sugar spike
3 p.m.	Handful of almonds and 4 pieces of chocolate	180	If you had had a complete breakfast this morning, you would not be reaching for chocolate; nuts are very high in fat. You should be eating a balanced meal here if you do not plan on having dinner until 8 p.m.
4 p.m.	Diet Coke; *I have one every afternoon*	Zero	Cola contains phosphates that have been shown to deplete bone mass.
6.30 p.m.	Quiznos veggie sub sandwich	230	If you had cheese and mayo, chances are that there is too much fat in the meal; this is also too low in protein ... not enough food.
9.45 p.m.	Extra-large chocolate chip cookie	210	A cookie is OK once in a while if it's eaten after a balanced meal, but alone it will not satisfy the body's needs.

Here is a one-day sample menu that I created for Nichole after she started the programme:

TIME OF MEAL	NICHOLE'S FOOD/ FEELING	CALORIES	CHRISTINE'S COMMENTS
Breakfast 7 a.m.	4 egg whites, 30 g (1 oz) low-fat veggie cheese, 225 g (7½ oz) pineapple, 1 slice multigrain bread spread with 100% natural fruit spread. *Feeling kinda full yet energized.*	310	Eaten within 1 hour of waking up. This meal is a good balance of proteins and high-fibre carbs, thus it will hold her over for approximately 4 hours.
Lunch 11 a.m.	Veggie cheese sandwich: 3 slices low-fat veggie cheese, cucumber, alfalfa sprouts, grated carrot, spinach, tomato, spread with avocado and low-fat cream cheese and a medium pear. *Lots of energy, and I'm in a good mood.*	410	Eaten 4 hours later, this is another fantastic healthy PC Combo. She will be satisfied until at least 3 p.m.
Lunch No. 2 3 p.m.	Edamame and lentil salad with brown rice and artichoke hearts (tinned in water), fat-free Italian dressing. *This was delicious and I'm surprised that I'm not craving sugar.*	410	Eaten 4 hours after the last meal. She is sure to be burning fat and saving muscle because her blood sugar is stable.
Dinner 7 p.m.	Low-fat tofu stir-fry – mixed veggies cooked with cooking spray, soy sauce and citrus juice – and a serving of brown rice. *This was good and I'm full; I can't even think of eating anything for the rest of the evening.*	330	Eaten 4 hours later. She will continue to have stable blood sugar levels and feel great throughout the evening.

'Before' meal totals: 1,810 calories, 82 grams protein, 271 grams carbs, 54 grams fat

'After' meal totals: 1,460 calories, 83 grams protein, 240 grams carbs, 21 grams fat

Nichole had been trying to lose 10 pounds (4½ kilograms) for 2 years with no success before she came to me. Her goal was to eat less and exercise more to lose weight, but her weight-loss strategy never worked because she was constantly hungry. As you see from her 'before' food log, her meals were not PC Combos and, thus, her blood sugar would constantly spike. She'd stay hungry all day without ever feeling satisfied.

Nichole suffered from lack of energy, caffeine cravings and mood swings, and her weight would not budge no matter what exercise or diet she tried. After we applied the ABCs to her eating habits, the stubborn fat began to melt away. In the beginning, Nikki was not happy about spending the extra time to cook and plan her food for each day, but after a few weeks she got the hang of it. She would come into my office perky and excited to share with me all of the new veggie proteins she had discovered. She created a shopping list of her favourite quick veggie protein/carb foods, and after she got into the routine of shopping and preparing her meals, it became a piece of cake. In the end, Nikki lost 12 pounds (5.4 kilograms) of body fat and maintained all of her muscle without eating one piece of meat. I believe she is an inspiration to vegetarians everywhere.

Short Protein List (for a more detailed protein list, see the Appendix)

EAT AS OFTEN AS YOU LIKE

- Chicken
- Turkey
- Fish (not including tuna, shark and swordfish)
- Egg whites
- Low-fat plain, regular or Greek yogurt
- Low-fat cottage cheese (low-salt is best)
- Low-fat ricotta cheese

- Other low-fat cheeses
- Prawns, scallops and shellfish
  (avoid if you have high cholesterol)
- Tempeh
- Beans and pulses

EAT UP TO FOUR TIMES PER WEEK

- Soya and tofu meals
- Tofu, firm
- Tofu, silken, firm (Mori-Nu)
- Edamame

EAT ONCE A WEEK

- Lean red meats (sirloin, tenderloin, any loin cut)
- Fish: tuna or mackerel – only one of either per week

EAT ONLY ONCE PER MONTH

- Swordfish or shark
- Lean pork

In Chapter 11, I'll show you dozens of ways to get more of these low-fat, high-protein foods into your diet. For now, just remember that you can't go wrong with any of the choices under 'Eat as Often as You Like', whether you're eating out or cooking for yourself.

Skinny Chick 10-Week Transformation

NAME: KATE B.

AGE: 27

TOTAL POUNDS LOST: 18 (8.2 kg)

TOTAL INCHES LOST: 27.75 (70 cm)

When I was younger, I was a gymnast, so I was always very muscular. As I got older, into secondary school, I wasn't involved in athletics and my eating habits were poor, so all of that bulk turned to fat.

I tried all the diets that everyone else has tried ... but there was something so unforgiving about those diets that I could only make it through a couple of weeks. I would get off track and never felt I could get back on.

The Skinny Chicks programme has so many positives. You feel great from the very beginning. Within a week, you feel a difference. Best of all, the programme is forgiving. I needed a programme that would help me to stay focused yet still live my life. During the course of the 10 weeks, I certainly found myself in a couple of situations where my food options were limited. In those cases, I would have whatever was being served, but I never felt that I was 'cheating', and I never felt that I couldn't get right back on the programme. I knew that my next meal was just 4 hours away, and I would get right back to eating a PC Combo.

When I walk out the door each morning, I take 60 seconds to go through what I'm going to be eating for the day, so there's a part of my life that's already planned out. I have control of that, and everything else falls into place from there.

It's really something when you're losing weight and you're eating properly – the power that you feel to achieve more. Christine had us focus on our dreams and goals outside health, and now I feel like everything's possible.

CHAPTER 8

The Carb Conspiracy

Carbohydrates are one of the most controversial subjects in the world of health and nutrition. It makes me angry when I hear people agree that you must reduce your carb intake to zero in order to lose weight. More than one celebrity client has stopped seeing me when I disagreed with this philosophy, and I have received ranting e-mails accusing me of being a pawn of the 'greedy corporations' who are promoting carbohydrates for profit. When an idea gets into people's minds, whether it's right or wrong, it is sometimes very hard to shake it loose. And of course we all know someone who lost a great deal of weight on an extreme low-carb diet – only to gain it back almost immediately. Today the tide is turning, but slowly; for almost 30 years many thousands of people swallowed this concept hook, line and sinker, and it's still part of today's nutritional landscape. Look in any supermarket and you can find a variety of products prominently labelled 'low carb' or 'no carb'. Bookshops are still loaded with low-carb and no-carb recipe books. Despite the fact that only a few years earlier, before low-carb became the dietary buzzword *du jour*, we were swept away by the 'low fat' diet fad and had managed to lose weight eating plenty of carbs, most people accepted the low-carb concept as gospel.

Many people, observing all the restaurant menus, books and supermarket products, assume that the people behind these offerings, with all their money and resources, must have access to the best scientific research. How could all those people be wrong? Not only that, several scientific studies, like the one published in the *Journal of the American Medical Association (JAMA)* in 2007 that compared the Atkins diet (low-carbohydrate), the Zone diet (40/30/40), the Ornish diet (low-fat) and a low-fat/high-carb diet amongst a group of women, reported that the Atkins diet resulted in the most rapid weight loss.

So there you have it: inarguable evidence validated by scientific studies. And you know what?

They are absolutely right.

If you stop eating carbs right now and simply eat all the steak, bacon, chicken, sausage, pork, turkey, eggs and dairy products you can find, you are going to lose weight – quickly. The science behind this is 100 per cent accurate. Sounds great, doesn't it? So why aren't we all Skinny Minnies by now?

As I said before, nutrition is never quite that simple. There are, of course, more than a few problems with this approach:

- When you don't supply your body with glucose from outside sources, it will try to get the glucose it needs from the glycogen in liver tissue and from the muscles themselves.

- Too much protein may cause kidney stones and aggravate existing kidney problems.

- A low-carb diet can result in the loss of calcium. One study showed that urinary calcium losses rose significantly in individuals following a low-carbohydrate, high–animal protein diet for 6 months. If you are not getting enough calcium from milk or a calcium supplement, your body will start to take it from your own bones, making them very weak and brittle.

- Somewhere between 1 to 3 days into such a diet, when your body may enter ketosis (see 'The Real Skinny on Ketosis'), you are truly breaking down fat for energy, but the breakdown is incomplete and there are several undesirable side effects.

- The worst problem, though, is not a matter of science but one of practical reality – most of us simply cannot stick to a low-carb

The Real Skinny on Ketosis

If you are familiar with the word *ketosis*, you have probably done some research into low-carb diets. Ketosis occurs when the body receives insufficient glucose during a fast or a low-carb diet. When glucose is not present, fat breakdown is incomplete and results in by-products known as ketone bodies. Your body is breaking down fat — but it is also breaking down muscle and other vital organs (this is, needless to say, a bad thing). Some of the undesirable side effects of ketosis include nausea, fatigue, bad breath and dizziness, and even worse, abnormal heart rhythms, calcium depletion, and liver and kidney problems.

Many people don't know about these side effects and believe that ketosis is a fantastic way to lose body fat. In the mid-1990s, during the height of my fitness modelling days, I was one of those people. I remember buying 'ketone strips' from the chemist. These were white strips of treated paper you urinated on; if they changed colour, that meant you had achieved ketosis. By the third day of limiting my carbs in order to achieve this state, I was half out of my mind, irrational, short-tempered, tired and confused. Worst of all, I had no idea I was actually slowing my metabolism and breaking down muscle tissue. I am grateful every day that I now know the Skinny Chicks programme is a much better way to lose fat!

diet. Ultimately, we cave in and binge on carbs to feed our starving bodies.

Speaking of reality, a closer look at the diet comparison study from *JAMA* reveals that few of the women actually stuck to their diets. Many on the non-Atkins diets were eating triple the amount of carbs they were supposed to eat. These women were in a scientific study conducted by top researchers at Stanford, a world-class university, and still they couldn't stick to their diets. What does that say for the rest of us? It says a lot.

When We Go on a Diet, Are We Really on a Diet?

The first thing we should all accept is that when we decide to go on a diet, the reality of what we eat is completely different from the diet we believe we are following. As you know from earlier chapters, I was just like the women in the *JAMA* study; I tried to keep from eating carbs, but the more I tried, the more my body would rebel and I would simply make up for the carb/energy deficit by overeating.

In fact, this was the subject of a segment I did for Rachael Ray's television talk show in the US. In this segment, two women had 1 whole week of eating videotaped. All of their food choices were recreated for the show, and the entire week of meals for each of these two brave women was laid out on a table for all the world to see. As the camera panned down the table from one day to the next, you could make out the same pattern. There would be a few 'dieting' days in a row, followed by a large binge day. After a binge day, most of us really starve ourselves – and these ladies were no different. But it was pretty shocking to see it laid out right before our eyes. And in reality, even on the days when they restricted their calories, there was always a cupcake, some cookies, a few glasses of wine or some kind of treat that the women just 'had to have'. Their eating was never consistent, and it was never really a diet. It was the same with me, and it is the same with the majority of my clients.

So . . . if we don't really diet when we diet, what should we be doing? How can we lose weight? The key is to avoid dieting altogether. A diet represents restriction and deprivation. As a nutritionist, my job is to make you healthier, and to do that, I need you to eat real food and real meals – carbs and all.

Gotta Have Carbs

My experience reviewing thousands of food journals for my clients confirms what we all know in our hearts: few of us can resist the urge to indulge in treats, most of them loaded with carbs. We live on Temptation Island, with carbs available everywhere, all the time. For some people, indulgence means a cookie here and there; for others it is a doughnut or two. For hard-core carbaholics like myself, it can mean eating a whole cake at one sitting. Your body will literally drag itself into the kitchen in the middle of the night to satisfy the carb urge. These urges are incredibly powerful.

When I read my clients' food journals, I can anticipate the carb binges. They usually take place after 2 or 3 days of limited carb consumption. After a few days of really small meals or protein-only meals, sure enough, the body makes up for the deficit as the person consumes a huge dinner followed by dessert, wine and a late-night treat. The lack of stable blood sugar – the result of consuming too many or too few carbs – causes the erratic eating that results in fat storage.

Let's look at the facts for a moment:

1. Our cells need carbs for the glucose fuel to live.

2. We live in a world where there are irresistible carbs everywhere.

3. Even when we go on a diet and say we will avoid carbs, we are going to eat some – or a lot.

4. These binges are driven by the body's need for carbs (and the hormonal imbalance created by erratic blood sugar levels).

5. If we were to eat a steady flow of healthy carbs with a lean protein, we would not be struck by these urges to binge.

6. The only way to eat for weight loss and better health is to eat balanced meals including protein, carbs and healthy fats every 4 hours.

I hope I have made my case.

Carbohydrates – the basics

The basic building blocks of carbohydrates are chains of sugar molecules. These sugar molecules are small enough to enter your bloodstream. By sugar molecules, I mean the same molecules that you sprinkle on your cornflakes. I know that bagels, pasta and bread don't taste like table sugar, but they are all made up of the same basic molecules.

You may have heard that it is better to have 'complex' rather than 'simple' carbs. Simple carbs are small sugar molecules that are easily digested and absorbed through the intestines. Complex carbs are just simple sugar molecules linked together; your body has to break the chain into simple sugar molecules that can enter the bloodstream. Because of this extra step, digestion of complex carbohydrates takes longer, which gives you a steadier supply of energy that is less likely to be converted into fat and stored. Examples of simple carbs are sugar, fruit, honey and maple syrup. Whole grains, potatoes and vegetables are complex carbs. But really, the more important question is how quickly a carb enters the bloodstream, and it turns out that you can't tell that just by knowing whether a particular food is a simple or complex carbohydrate.

How the Glycaemic Index Confuses the Issue

At one time it was thought that simple carbs were 'bad' because they caused a spike in blood sugar, while complex carbs were 'good' because they provided a steadier release of glucose that kept blood sugar stable. As it turns out, however, not all simple carbs are bad and not all complex carbs are good. In the 1980s, researchers developed what was thought to be a better way to identify the good from the bad. It's called the glycaemic index (GI). Simply put, the glycaemic index is a number given to carbs to reflect the rate at which they cause glucose levels in the blood to rise; the higher a carb's glycaemic index rating, the faster it converts to glucose in the blood. Carbs with a GI of 55 or less cause only a tiny rise; those in the 55 to 70 range cause levels to rise a bit more; and carbs with GIs above 70 cause blood glucose levels to spike. For example, a baked potato has a GI level of 85 (big spike) and a sweet potato has a GI level of 54 (little blip); a baguette has a GI of 85, while an apple has a GI of 36; and pre-cooked rice has a GI of 90, while brown rice has a GI of 55.

As you may already have guessed, high-GI carbs get the 'bad' carb rap. Indeed, a meal that consists only of high-GI carbs will cause insulin levels to soar, pushing glucose into cells only to cause your blood sugar levels to fall lower than before you ate. You'll be hungry again and may find yourself at the vending machine desperate for that bag of M&Ms. Meanwhile, that

The Real Skinny
on Eating by Numbers

It's not realistic to think you can live by assigning a number to every carb you eat. Bowl of strawberries: 32. Oat biscuit: 55. Melba toast: 70. Not to mention, those numbers can be deceiving: the GI of cornflakes is in the 80s, while a Snickers bar clocks in at 61! And carrots and watermelon both have off-the-chart GI readings; however, both are composed mostly of water and fibre and are chock full of nutrients – they actually contain only a very small amount of carbs. Going strictly by the numbers, you would miss out on those two healthy and delicious food choices.

Two of the worst offenders, according to the GI, are white rice and baked potatoes. Bear in mind, though, that these measurements are taken on the food in its pure state, with nothing added. Let me ask you this – have you ever eaten a bare baked potato in your whole lifetime? I think not. Putting butter on your baked potato will actually improve the GI (make it lower) because the fat in the butter basically introduces more traffic to the Blood Sugar Freeway and lowers the GI. Now don't think you can melt a large knob of butter and a massive dollop of soured cream onto your baked potato; you don't want to put the fat content through the roof just to lower the GI. However, you can stuff that potato with some low-fat Cheddar cheese and broccoli . . . now we're talkin'!

overload of insulin contributes to your weight gain by stashing excess glucose into fat cells. And remember, high insulin levels also prevent fat cells from releasing stored energy when your body needs it. When you want to lose weight, you want those body fat storage cells to give up their stored energy; the more energy they pay out, the better your chances of successfully zipping up your 'skinny' jeans. By contrast, a plate of low-GI carbs raises blood sugar slowly and steadily. Insulin levels rise only high enough to gently nudge glucose into waiting cells, where it is burned for energy, and your blood sugar stays steady for hours. Research shows that when your blood sugar is steady, you feel satisfied and full. That bag of M&Ms will stay in the vending machine to tempt another.

There are dozens of sites on the Internet and many books that will give you the GI value of any given food, should you wish to know. But, as with everything else we've been discussing, it isn't quite that simple. The GI is a measurement taken in a laboratory where the food is isolated. In real life, we almost always eat foods together with other foods. We hardly ever eat cereal without milk or rice without a main course. The best news is that when you eat a PC Combo, you lower the GI of any carb since the protein (and the healthy fats) will slow traffic on the Blood Sugar Freeway.

It's Not All about the Numbers

Here's how the GI can be deceiving. Doughnuts, jellybeans, cupcakes, Pop Tarts, Skittles and Coca-Cola all have a lower GI than a plain baked potato, yet clearly none of these are healthy food choices. Chemically speaking, you could eat a grilled chicken breast with jellybeans and your body would be receiving the balance of protein and carbs that it needs to keep blood sugar stable. But this jellybean meal will not make you feel as full and healthy as the same grilled chicken breast eaten with a baked potato and low-fat soured cream. The jellybean feast is less substantial and not as wholesome, and you will simply not feel good after you eat it. If you've ever been a yo-yo dieter (and who hasn't?), you've experienced the difference in how your body feels after a healthy meal and after an unhealthy one. That feeling of well-being you get after a nutritious meal is crucial because without it, you will be much more tempted to grab that extra doughnut or drink that large sugary coffee.

Use your common sense. If you're going to use the GI to choose foods, use it intelligently. For instance, natural sweeteners include sugar, honey and agave nectar (a natural liquid sweetener extracted from the agave plant). Sugar has a GI of about 58; honey, because it comes from a variety of sources, can vary from about 32 to 80; and agave's GI is between 11 and 19. Several of the recipes in this book use agave nectar. That doesn't mean I never use honey – I especially like the taste of honey in my tea.

Any whole food (e.g. watermelon) is going to be a healthier choice than a food that is made of a variety of ingredients including chemical preservatives (e.g. ice cream or jellybeans). You don't want to overdo either of these foods, but watermelon (an excellent source of potassium, lycopene, and vitamins A, C and B_6) will certainly leave you feeling healthier than ice cream. So don't just go down the GI list and choose a low number for your carbs. Instead, choose a healthy carbohydrate to eat with your lean protein at every meal.

The Perils of the Lonely Carb

Many experts recommend the consumption of whole grain cereals and breads, steel-cut or pinhead (Scotch) oats, wholewheat pasta and beans while discouraging potatoes. I completely agree that these are great healthy choices. But on the Skinny Chicks programme, you have the option of eating potatoes, white rice and pasta, should you want them, *as long as* they are accompanied by a lean protein and a healthy fat. Otherwise, you will definitely cause your blood sugar to rise and fall dramatically. Generally speaking, the best way to consume a carb is in a state as close to its natural, fresh-off-the-plant form as possible. The more you chop it, grind it, wash it and bleach it, the less time it takes for your body to break it down into a simple sugar molecule. For instance, wheat starts out as a whole grain, is then stripped of its outer layer (where most of the nutrients live), and is eventually processed and bleached and filled with preservatives until we see it on the supermarket shelf as part of a loaf of white bread. A whole apple is digested more slowly than stewed apple, which is digested more slowly than apple juice. All of these must always be combined with a lean, healthy protein at every meal to cause plenty of traffic on the Blood Sugar Freeway.

When you begin the Skinny Chicks eating plan, you will only eat superhealthy carbs and PC Combos for the first 2 weeks. This gets your weight loss off to a nice, quick, healthy start. I call this phase, appropriately, the kick-start. Then, later, you will incorporate all your favourite carbs into your eating plan for life. This will give you the freedom to live and enjoy life without giving up your favourite foods (most of them, anyway).

Skinny Chick 10-Week Transformation

NAME: JEANNE M.

AGE: 53

TOTAL POUNDS LOST: 18 (8.2 kg)

TOTAL INCHES LOST: 20.75 (70 cm)

When I turned 40, I felt like I was cursed with the fat gene. The forties were all about the 'F' words for me: fat, flabby, frumpy. I just kept putting on weight and I couldn't get it off. I tried everything to get my metabolism working again and even hired a personal trainer, but nothing was happening. I kept putting on weight and I was very frustrated – another 'F' word. Then I found out about the Skinny Chicks programme.

Now that I'm in my fifties, and I've been following the Skinny Chicks programme, there are some more 'F' words – but this time it's 'fabulous'. I feel 'fantastic'. I'm 'firming' up and I feel 'faster' at everything I do.

Before I started the programme, I had bad eating habits. I didn't know that I needed to combine carbohydrates with protein. I was one of those people who bought into the whole no-carb diet. I lost weight quickly, but it would come back on and it wouldn't come off again. When I started combining proteins with carbohydrates and eating four times a day as Christine advised me, I dropped a size in 3 weeks. Then I dropped another dress size after 6 weeks on the programme. I have more weight to lose, but I am on the fast track to losing a lot more weight and getting back into shape.

CHAPTER 9

The Fat
Fear Factor

I once saw the late comedian Sam Kinison perform his stand-up routine. Near the end, he got all quiet and sensitive. In a soft, caring voice, he said, 'You women, if there is something you want us men to do, any little things that we can do to make you happy . . . ' He paused for a moment, then yelled as only he could, 'THEN WHY DON'T YOU GIVE US SOME POSSIBLE CLUE WHAT THE HECK IT IS???!!! TELL US!!!!! WE'LL DO IT!!!' It is hard to convey in writing how funny Sam was, but his point was this: don't make me guess – just keep it simple. People losing weight have the same plea: just tell me what not to eat. Fewer carbs? Fine. Less fat? No problem.

Before carbs were singled out as dietary villains, the 'low-fat' approach was often touted as the best way to lose weight. Soon dieters were munching guiltlessly on fat-free cookies, fat-free ice cream and fat-free salad dressing. The theory was as simple as it gets: to *be* less fat, *eat* less fat.

So what happened? We Westerners got fatter and fatter, that's what happened. All those food manufacturers who jumped on the fat-free bandwagon forgot to remind us that fat free does not mean calorie free. And we consumers, thinking we had found the once-and-for-all, final-answer, easy way to lose weight, did not stop to read the labels of the foods we were buying.

We now know that we need fats just as we need carbs. We just don't need as many fats as most of us consume.

Skinny Chicks (a.k.a. healthy people) should understand what's up with fat, and what fat does on the inside of the body as well as the outside. Fats are an important subject, and this chapter will review and explain the various types and functions of fats, when they are appropriate and why it's not a good idea to cut fats completely out of your diet repertoire.

Meet Joleen, Who Had No Idea

A few years ago I worked with a mother of three small children, who told me I came highly recommended by some of her fellow school mums. Joleen was smart, well-educated and very active chasing after her toddlers every day. Despite her activity level and some extreme dieting, she could not shed the baby weight from her third child. Joleen told me that losing her pregnancy weight after the first two children had been really easy because she would just restrict carbohydrates and exercise, and the weight would simply come off. But not this time around.

The first thing I asked Joleen to do was to keep a 24-hour food journal the day before our first consultation appointment, which is my usual procedure for new clients. When Joleen arrived at my office, I performed my standard tests: body fat analysis using digital skin fold calipers, body composition test (also to measure body fat) using bioelectrical impedance, girth measurements and blood sugar analysis. I calculated the amount of body fat versus lean tissue. Her body fat percentage was 28 per cent. As a reference, anything over 25 per cent for an adult woman is considered overweight, while 30 per cent body fat is considered obese. Joleen was shocked because she was a US size 8 (UK size 10) and did not feel like she had high body fat. I explained to her that most women who come into my office start out at about 33 per cent body fat, which made her body fat percentage actually lower than my average client. I went on to tell her that when I first began my nutrition certification programme, I actually started out at 28 per cent body fat myself, even though I was an avid exerciser and low-carb dieter at the time.

Next, I reviewed her food journal and immediately saw that for breakfast she was consuming 22 grams of fat, most of it saturated. She used a knob of butter (10 grams of fat) to fry her two eggs (8 grams of fat). For a mid-morning snack she would consume two handfuls of nuts (30 grams of fat) and for lunch she would have a big salad (surprise!) with lots of meat, green leaves and 4 to 6 tablespoons of dressing (approximately 42 grams of fat). So, by lunchtime, this mother of three had consumed 84 grams of fat! That is twice my recommended fat intake for a full day. Her afternoon snack was either two full-fat cheese cubes (15 grams of fat) or two handfuls of nuts (30 grams of fat). Finally, her dinner was grilled, roasted or pan-fried meat served with steamed vegetables with one or two knobs of butter. I informed her that her daily intake of fat was approximately 120 grams (I recommend around 40 grams per day). That is 1,080 calories from fat. Her daily caloric intake, including fat and protein, added up to 2,100 calories.

Joleen was shocked to realize how much fat she was consuming. Nor had she realized that it was mostly artery-clogging saturated fat. I told her she was not alone, and that many women were eating this way because they had experienced rapid weight loss during the first few weeks of low-carb diets. However, for most women there comes a time when the weight loss stops and the body decides enough is enough. That's where the Skinny Chicks programme comes in.

I explained to Joleen that she *should* eat fat, and that fat is good for her, but that to lose weight, most women need to eat no more than 10 to 13 grams of fat per meal (even less if you have a small frame). I got her to incorporate healthy, high-fibre carbohydrates, lean proteins and healthy fats into each meal. After only 1 week on my programme she came into my office and I weighed her. She had lost 4 pounds (1.8 kilograms) – a good week. But I knew that Joleen, who had been such a die-hard low-carb advocate, might have a hard time taking my advice about eating a balance of protein, carbs and fats. Often, low-carb advocates pay me for my advice but then they simply go on a super-strict zero-carb diet. So I didn't want to get too excited until I did her body fat test. If she'd lost 4 pounds of muscle, it would mean she'd restricted carbs (restricting carbs for a week will cause the body to burn lots of muscle tissue). But if the 4 pounds she had lost were from body fat, I would know that she had cut back on fat intake and added in some healthy carbs. I did her body fat test and, sure enough, she was down 1 per cent body fat, which means that she lost 4 pounds of fat in only 1 week! Joleen was delighted to be losing body fat and losing it from her waist first. With these quick results, she continued on my programme and lost all of her extra baby weight in 6 weeks, for a total weight loss of 12 pounds (5.4 kilograms) of fat. She is now back to the weight and size she was on her wedding day. To this day, she comes to my office every 4 months just to check in and have me test her body fat. Joleen is so excited about what she learned on my programme that I receive referrals from her constantly. All these women are very successful on my programme, and I believe that mums are some of my most special clients because they are passing down their nutrition habits to their precious little ones . . . the children.

Fast Fat Facts

The reality is that for weight loss, it still is and always will be important to reduce excess dietary fat intake. Why? Because fat in your food can translate into fat on your tummy, bum, thighs, arms or anywhere your body fat tends to accumulate. Here is how it happens: of the three energy-yielding nutrients (proteins, carbohydrates and fats), fats contain the most energy/calories per gram. By now you probably know that both protein and carbohydrates have 4 calories per gram, while fat has 9 calories per gram. When we eat too much, it doesn't matter what we are eating, our bodies can and will convert it to fat storage. But the metabolic pathway from dietary fat to body fat requires the fewest steps when compared with carbohydrate and protein breakdown. Fat goes from lips to hips more easily than any other nutrient. This is one of the reasons I recommend limiting daily fat intake to 20 per cent of your overall caloric intake. Too much of a good thing is never good . . . right?

For many of my clients, the whole low-fat-no-fat fiasco has caused a great deal of confusion and frustration. It's important to clear up this misunderstanding; in fact, it's a matter of life and death. So here goes:

All bodily cells need fats to function. Fats provide fuel for cells. They also provide raw materials for building cell membranes and the outer layer that surrounds the cell and controls what goes in and out of the cell itself. Fats also create protective sheaths that surround nerves. Fats are the building blocks for some hormones as well as for chemicals that control muscle contractions and blood clotting. The body can make most of the fats it needs from any fat in the diet or from carbohydrates. However, there are a small number of fats your body needs that cannot be created within the body. These are called essential fats, and they only come from the foods we eat. That's why it's not only unnecessary to avoid fat in your diet, it's vital that you include it. However, just as with carbs, all fats are not created equal. In total, there are four kinds of fat: one you should make an effort not to overdo, one you should avoid like the plague and two that are must-haves.

The 'Bad' Fats

- **Saturated fats:** These are generally solid at room temperature and come mainly from animals and animal products such as whole milk, cream, butter, cheese, red meat and palm oil. Why are these fats bad for you? To begin with, saturated fats cause LDL ('bad') levels of cholesterol to rise, because they prevent cholesterol from getting inside the cells. (Cholesterol is not all bad – it is required for the formation of bile acids, which are needed for fat digestion; it is used to make important hormones such as oestrogen and progesterone; and it is involved in the formation of vitamin D in the skin.) That leaves excess cholesterol floating around in the bloodstream, where it can become part of the plaque that builds up in your arteries. According to the UK government Department of Health heart disease is the biggest killer in the country, killing more than 110,000 people in England alone every year. The number one suspect in heart disease is saturated fat.

  However, here is something you must understand. Saturated

fats have their good points. They are a good source of energy when our bodies are low on fuel; they act as 'shock absorbers' for our internal organs; and they insulate us from the cold. Saturated fats are only harmful when they're consumed in excess. One little knob of butter will not do you in – but great gobs of it on a stack of pancakes every Sunday will probably clog your arteries. Experts recommend choosing fats and oils with predominantly unsaturated fatty acids – see the 'Good' Fats, below.

- **Trans fats:** Trans fat is vegetable oil that has been heated in the presence of hydrogen gas and nickel oxide, in a process known as partial hydrogenation. That transforms vegetable oil into solid fat. This explains how we get margarine and products such as Stork, which was introduced as a branded product in 1920. In the UK there is no requirement for the labelling of trans fats on food labels, but some manufacturers have started to do so voluntarily.

Manufacturers love trans fats because they extend the shelf life of food, but too much trans fat in your diet will cut *your* shelf life short. Trans fat is worse for you than saturated fat; it can raise bad LDL cholesterol and lower good HDL cholesterol and has been linked to both heart disease and diabetes. Putting trans fats into your body is like dropping grains of sand into a Swiss watch; sooner or later, it will stop working. Trans fats will cause arteries to clog up and eventually contribute to heart attacks and strokes, so it is a good idea to find foods that are cooked without them. They are so harmful that New York City, in a move that made history, banned trans fats from all city restaurants. You can avoid trans fats by staying away from fast foods and by reading the labels of packaged goods. Anything that contains hydrogenated vegetable oil or partially hydrogenated vegetable oil should be put back unopened where it can sit and live out its shelf life alone and untouched. And don't be fooled by 'diet' foods like protein bars and low-fat ice cream; they may contain trans fats as well.

The 'Good' Fats

- **Monounsaturated fats:** These fats are liquid at room temperature, but start to solidify at refrigerator temperature. They come from certain plant oils, including olive, rapeseed (canola) and peanut oils, as well as avocado. Eat up!

- **Polyunsaturated fats:** These fats are liquid at room temperature and in the fridge. You'll find polyunsaturated fats in seeds and in oils made from corn, soya, sesame, safflower and sunflower, as well as in nuts and fish. Replacing the saturated fats in your diet with unsaturated fats may help lower your blood cholesterol level. However, before you go out and fill yourself up with fat (unsaturated or otherwise), remember this: fat contains more than twice the calories of either protein or carbohydrate. You only need a small amount – 10–15 grams – of healthy fat in every meal, always eaten as part of a PC Combo, of course.

The 'Superhero' Fats

If you're looking for the fats your body needs to save the day (as far as your health is concerned), you'll call on the superhero of the fat world: omega-3s.

Both omega-3s and omega-6s are essential fatty acids (EFAs), necessary for human health. Our bodies can't produce EFAs, so we must get them from the foods we eat. Omega-3 is typically found in oily fish, flaxseed (linseed) and walnuts. Omega-6 is found in corn, soya, rapeseed (canola), safflower and sunflower oil. A balance of these two fats is necessary for optimal health. Unfortunately, most Westerners consume a far larger number of omega-6s than omega-3s, and this is a problem, as an imbalance may contribute to serious health problems. That means you should try to include more sources of omega-3 in your diet.

There are three main omega-3 fatty acids found in the diet. The first two are eicosapentaenoic acid (EPA) and docosahexaenoic acid (DHA) Also known as long-chain omega-3s, they are found mostly in coldwater fish, including salmon, trout, fresh tuna, mackerel, sea bass, herring, oysters and sardines. The third omega-3 is alpha-linolenic acid (ALA) and comes from plant sources including flaxseed (linseed), walnuts, sunflower seeds, rapeseed (canola) oils, soya, wheat germ and dark leafy greens. Some of the many benefits of omega-3s include:

- **Weight loss.** EFAs help improve insulin sensitivity, help prevent type 2 diabetes and help keep your blood sugar stable, which, as we know, is essential for weight loss and maintenance. Fats in the bloodstream help slow down the speed at which glucose flows. EFAs also increase your body's metabolic rate and help burn fat. Does this mean you can eat a ton of fat with your carbs? No; not if you want to have a fit and lean body. Think of fats as a small flavoursome helper, but not your primary fuel.

  One interesting study from the University of South Australia showed that women who ate fish or took fish oil supplements and exercised lost more weight than those who did either one alone. The study's researchers believe that the fatty acids in fish oils activate enzymes that enhance the fat-burning effects of exercise.

- **Heart health.** Omega-3s are polyunsaturated, so they don't cause plaque buildup in the arteries that can lead to heart disease. A 2006 study from Harvard University determined that 250 milligrams a day of DHA and EPA from fish or fish oil supplements helped reduce the risk of dying from a heart attack by 36 per cent.

- **Joint health.** Omega-3s have been shown to decrease the production of inflammatory proteins called cytokines, which are known to play a role in stripping cartilage and eroding bone. And studies have shown that people who consume fish oils have fewer tender joints and decreased stiffness.

- **Mood lifter.** The US National Institutes of Health has stated that two 115-g (4-ounce) servings of fatty fish, such as salmon, halibut or tinned light tuna, per week may significantly raise your levels of serotonin, a mood-boosting brain chemical. Other studies have shown that people who live in countries with higher rates of fish consumption have lower rates of clinical depression, bipolar disorder and postnatal depression. Not only that, people who consumed higher levels of EPA and DHA were less likely to report feeling 'blue'. Dr Bill Sears, associate clinical professor of paediatrics at the University of California, told the *Los Angeles Times* in May 2008, 'There's a lot of good science on food and the brain, particularly in the area of omega-3 fatty acids. In fact, the first so-called medicine I prescribe for a child with any type of learning, behaviour or mood disorder is high doses of omega-3.'

● **Cognitive improvement.** Your mother was right; fish is brain food. EFAs are essential to brain health. The brain is made up of 60 per cent fat. Diets that are too low in fat can have serious cognitive consequences. On the other hand, studies have shown that people who eat fish two or three times per week are half as likely to experience age-related cognitive decline, including Alzheimer's disease.

● **Great skin and shiny hair.** You may be able to tell a person who is deficient in fatty acids because they will have dry, flaky skin, dandruff and eczema. EFAs help your skin maintain its elasticity and youthful glow, and they help keep hair healthy and shiny.

The recommendation in the UK is that to get the maximum benefit adults and children over 12 are advised to eat two portions of fish per week (a portion is about 145 grams/5 ounces, cooked weight), one of which should be oily. If you are not able to do that, you should take an omega-3 supplement for the many benefits.

Nuts about Nuts

Many experts recommend a handful of nuts if you are hungry, because, they say, nuts are a great source of protein. However, I teach my clients to think of nuts as a 'good fat' and not a protein. If you look at the nutrition facts for nuts, you will see that nuts are much higher in fat than in protein. And considering the fact that fat in our foods converts

The Real Skinny on ALA

Alpha-linolenic acid (ALA) is a type of plant-derived omega-3 fatty acid that has many of its own benefits. It has been shown to reduce the risk of total cholesterol, lower LDL (bad) cholesterol, help lower blood pressure and keep platelets from becoming sticky, thus reducing the risk of a heart attack. A 16-year study from Harvard University of nearly 77,000 female nurses found that women with the highest intake of ALA (1.5 grams per day) had a 46 per cent lower risk of sudden cardiac death than those who consumed only 0.7 gram per day. I find the easiest way to ensure that I'm getting my fair share of ALA is to sprinkle some ground flaxseed (linseed) on top of my cereal or porridge in the morning, or on yogurt for a snack, or to add it to delicious fruit smoothies.

into fat on our bodies, I cannot tell clients to use nuts as a protein source if they need to lose weight. If you are at your optimal weight and your metabolism is healthy, by all means ignore me and go nuts! But for myself and everyone on the Skinny Chicks programme, I say consider nuts a 'good fat'.

Many diets also recommend nut butters, such as peanut butter, almond butter and macadamia butter. But these are also inadequate protein sources. I constantly see new clients in my office who truly believe that by spreading peanut butter on their morning toast, they are getting loads of protein. Sadly, they are getting a double dose of fat (healthy fat but still fat) and a single dose of an incomplete protein (non–animal based proteins often do not offer all nine essential amino acids; thus they are called incomplete proteins). Spreading peanut butter on wholemeal toast would technically give you a complete protein, but you're still getting a double dose of fat.

Read the chart on the opposite page, and look closely at the grams of protein and grams of fat in each; you will notice there is about twice as much fat as there is protein in most types of nuts and nut butters.

FOOD	SERVING SIZE	PROTEIN (G)	FAT (G)
Almonds	60 g (2 oz)	12.5	30
Almond butter	2 tbsp	5	18
Brazil nuts	60 g (2 oz)	8	38
Cashews	60 g (2 oz)	9	26
Cashew butter	2 tbsp	5	14
Hazelnuts	60 g (2 oz)	8	34
Macadamia nuts	60 g (2 oz)	4	43
Peanuts	60 g (2 oz)	13	28
Peanut butter	2 tbsp	7	16
Pecans	60 g (2 oz)	5	42
Pine nuts	60 g (2 oz)	8	39
Pistachios	60 g (2 oz)	12	26
Sunflower seeds	60 g (2 oz)	11	20
Walnuts	60 g (2 oz)	14	33

Here are the exceptions:

Soya nuts	60 g (2 oz)	21	13
Soya nut butter	2 tbsp	7	11

Perhaps even more importantly, neither a handful of nuts nor a few tablespoons of nut butter will satisfy your hunger the way a serving of the lean proteins beginning on page 287 will. I have clients who are in tears because they are so tired of being hungry. A handful of nuts is not enough, and they end up overeating later in the day to make up for it. So stop driving yourself nuts with the notion that nuts will facilitate weight loss, because they seldom do.

Skinny Chick 10-Week Transformation

NAME: JENNIFER H.

AGE: 46

TOTAL POUNDS LOST: 14 (6.4 kg)

TOTAL INCHES LOST: 25.5 (64.8 cm)

I was one of those people who was always very skinny. Even when I put on weight, I felt that I was skinny. But when I reached my forties and was going through the perimenopause, I put on about 1 stone 6 pounds (9 kilograms). For the past 10 years, I've been on many different diets, and I would lose 5 or 10 pounds (2¼ or 4½ kilograms), but I'd never feel good about it and would always put it right back on.

With Christine's Skinny Chicks programme, there were two really cool things. I had accumulated this belly fat, which I absolutely hated. Her programme is the first one of all the nutrition plans I encountered where the belly fat came off first. In addition, I lost weight on my legs, and that feels great, too. You're not just losing weight on the scales, you're also losing inches. And your body shape changes. It's amazing. Even my clothes from when I was thinner don't fit any more because the whole body changes on the Skinny Chicks programme. You really lengthen everything, and you get strong and lean and you lose all that excess fat.

What surprised me were the other benefits I got from the programme. I've suffered from migraine headaches my whole life. In recent years, I've been taking a prescription medicine plus painkillers all the time. I was at the point where I was getting four to six migraines a month. I have two teenagers, I own a business and I just don't have time for that kind of illness. However, since the second week of the Skinny Chicks programme, I haven't had one migraine. I think that is just a miracle.

I grew up in the fast-food generation. We're all busy and on the go all the time. But what I've learned is that even on the go, you can eat healthily. I learned not to let myself get to the point where I'm starving, to eat combinations of carbs and proteins, and to make sure I'm not eating a lot of processed foods. As Christine says, if you can't read it, you probably shouldn't eat it.

I have two teenage girls, and it's very important to me that they don't see me on some fad diet because I want to set a good example for them. On the Skinny Chicks programme, we all tend to eat healthy meals together.

This programme has made me realize that no matter what point you're at in your life, you can still always learn something and get remotivated. I feel great, I look great and it permeates into other parts of my life.

Skinny Chick Chat

DEAR CHRISTINE: One of the reasons I never succeed on a diet is that I'm usually hungry all the time. This drives me crazy (just ask my friends and family). What can I do to lose weight without being hungry all day?

ROSEMARY T.

ROSEMARY: That is one of the greatest things about my programme. Rather than depriving yourself, you get to eat real meals every 4 hours. Since you are eating this often and the meals are a balance of protein, carbs and some healthy fats, you won't feel hungry until it is time for your next meal. Remember — try to keep healthy fats down to 10 grams of fat per meal and eat them with the rest of your meal, rather than alone as you would a handful of nuts. I think you will be much more satisfied and happier.

EAT WELL, CHRISTINE

CHAPTER 10

Drink Yourself Skinny

When I was a teenager, one of my first jobs was at Baskin-Robbins the ice cream parlour. (Hey, I needed some way to pay for my Duran Duran albums.) But Baskin-Robbins has recently distinguished itself in nutrition infamy. In March 2008, the US edition of *Men's Health* magazine ranked the Baskin-Robbins large Heath Bar Shake as the 'unhealthiest drink in America', no small achievement. At 2,310 calories and with 108 grams of fat (64 of them 'bad' saturated fats), this drink is destined to take up permanent residence on your buttocks and around your middle. It weighs in at 6 times my recommended caloric intake for a single meal and 11 times the fat. If you ate an otherwise balanced diet, but drank one of these each day, you could go from skinny to fat in a few weeks with no effort. The only people who should ever drink these are actors trying to bulk up to play overweight characters, which is a world market of about 10 people. (Even for them, I would recommend something without so much saturated fat.) Sorry, Baskin-Robbins – I appreciate your giving me the job when I needed it, but I can't recommend your shake.

The market is now awash with delicious but horrifically unhealthy drinks. In 2007, a panel of experts on nutrition and health estimated that about 21 per cent of calories consumed by Americans over the age of 2 come from beverages, especially soft drinks and fruit drinks with added sugar. Compounding the problem, the panel found, is that beverages have 'weak satiety properties' – they don't fill you up or curb your appetite – and people do not compensate for the beverage calories by eating less food.

Even flavoured waters aren't 'free' food. They taste great and provide vitamins, right? Well, maybe so, but they also contain about 120 calories per bottle – still more than you should be taking in between meals. Look at it this way: if you drink two 'healthy' Vitamin Waters per day in addition to your usual calorie intake, you could put on 1 pound (4.5 kilograms) in 14½ days!

OK, so what number is low enough? What is the right number of calories in a drink?

Zilch. Nada. Zero. Not one. If you want to slim down, you should not be getting a single calorie from your drinks.

What you should be drinking is water. Every doctor, every diet and every nutrition plan says you need to drink at least 8 glasses of water every day. I agree – your body needs a lot of fresh water every day. What's confusing us now are the hundreds of varieties of water or 'water-type' beverages available in every supermarket and corner shop.

It's extremely important to make the distinction between a sugary drink and water. You might look at a bottle and think, 'Hey, I know I need 8 glasses of water per day; why not make it a great-tasting drink? This drink is mostly water, but better tasting, and the label says it includes loads of vitamins (or antioxidants or other "health benefits").' So instead of drinking water, you might choose to sip on a sweet drink all day long. When you do this every day, it really adds up. So before you buy that 'healthy' watery drink, make sure you read the label to see what you're really getting.

What about Juice?

Nearly everybody knows by now that all the sugar and harmful ingredients in fizzy drinks are not going to help you lose weight. But what about fruit juices? Aren't they a good source of vitamins, minerals and

The Real Skinny on Losing Water

Your body must excrete a minimum of 480 millilitres (16 fluid ounces) of water per day as urine to carry away metabolic waste. We also lose water through breathing and sweating. When performing cardiovascular exercise, an adult can sweat off 1.5 litres (2½ pints) of fluid in 1 hour. For most people, the average daily water loss is approximately 2½ litres (4½ pints) per day. We need about 120 millilitres (4 fluid ounces) of water for every 100 calories expended. For most people, that is about 2 to 3 litres of water (3½ to 5 pints) per day.

phytonutrients? Yes, they are, but they are also loaded with sugar in the form of fructose. Drinking even natural fruit juices between meals is simply pouring sugar into your bloodstream. As we learned, this can lead to storage of body fat. However, having a small glass of juice with a meal is fine as long as you recognize the juice as part of your carbo-hydrate portion. But for best results, I recommend you stick to zero-calorie beverages during your weight loss phase unless otherwise specified in the Skinny Chicks meal plan.

What happens if you drink fruit juice (or any other sugary drink) all day long? Remember the fuel tanks we learned about in Chapter 3? If you're drinking sugar all day, Tank 1 (blood sugar) will always be full and you will never reach Tank 2 (glycogen in the liver and muscle tissue plus body fat), and thus you'll never burn any body fat.

Now let's look at the caloric cost of drinking juice instead of water with meals. One medium-size glass of orange juice contains about 150 calories. Suppose you started drinking one glass each day with break-fast and did nothing else differently. In the course of a year, you would put on about 16 pounds, but you wouldn't feel any fuller because juice is just liquid. If you simply swapped that glass of juice for water, you would theoretically lose 1 stone 2 pounds (7.2 kilograms) in a year with-out feeling any hungrier or expending any additional effort.

However, there is a big difference between theory and reality. Yes, your body can get the water it needs either way, but the orange juice contains a lot of energy in the form of sugar. If you cut that out, your body will subconsciously reach for a few more bites to compensate for the lost energy of the orange juice. This might come in the form of a bag of potato crisps or an extra scoop of rice, or maybe a few more bites of dessert at night. In theory, you simply change the juice for water, but in reality your body compensates.

So does that mean that all hope is lost? Of course not. Here is the plan:

1. Drink chilled water all day long between meals to keep your body hydrated (I highly recommend you add some lemon slices to your ice water for the added flavour, the spa-like feel and the antioxidant benefits).

2. If you want to drink fruit juice, have it with meals and be sure to keep the overall amounts of protein, carbs, and healthy fats in balance.

3. In moderation (no more than two or three times per week), you can drink a diet cola or another zero-calorie drink.

It is as simple as that.

Coffee Breaks: I'll Take a Direct Injection, Please

Everybody needs to take a coffee break now and then, and I don't have a real issue with coffee or even caffeine. Caffeine, when taken to excess, can interfere with the function of the adrenal system and the nervous system. But research studies have shown that a single cup of coffee each day will not harm you and can increase clarity of mind and alertness (thank goodness).

The problem is that you don't go to the espresso bar for a regular filter coffee. You want something creamy, dreamy and delicious. I strongly believe that the innovation of high-calorie beverages, including coffee drinks, is a major cause of our increasing obesity rates. Most patrons of these coffee joints are ordering lattes, caramel macchiatos and frappuccinos – all of which are very high in calories and fats. To make matters worse, many people add a huge dollop of whipped cream on top.

A venti frappuccino with whipped cream from Starbucks in the US packs in almost 600 calories – almost 50 per cent more than I recommend for a full meal. But a frappuccino is definitely *not* a meal. It briefly postpones your appetite for lunch or dinner, but it doesn't fill you up or satisfy you.

This doesn't mean you need to steer clear of Starbucks altogether. There are several great zero-calorie drinks that you can order at your favourite coffee shop. The very best order, hands down, is green tea. Green tea is a natural fat burner due to its thermogenic properties, which enhance fatty acid oxidation. Green tea is also loaded with anti-oxidants called catechins that are thought to help with weight loss. In one study, metabolic rate was increased by an average of 266 calories per day, which means you could lose approximately 1 pound (450 grams) every 2 weeks simply by drinking 8 to 10 cups of tea (or by taking a 90-milligram green tea extract supplement). Green tea also has an amino acid in it called L-theanine, which boosts alpha brain waves and promotes alert relaxation, and who doesn't need a little of that each day? In addition to its weight loss and cognitive benefits, tea contains anti-cancer agents and reduces the risk of heart disease, high blood pressure, tooth decay and even bad breath. With all the wonderful benefits of tea, I highly recommend that you get into the habit of ordering green tea (or any tea – white, green, oolong or black) during your daily coffee run.

If you can't make the transition to tea, the next best things to order are espressos, Americanos and regular filter coffees. All are nearly calorie-free and won't interfere with your metabolism or appetite. As soon as you start adding milk to your drink, even skimmed milk, you are consuming calories, altering your meal schedule and keeping your body from dipping into Tank 2 (always burning blood sugar for fuel, never

Skinny Chick 10-Week Transformation

NAME: JOY L.

AGE: 48

TOTAL POUNDS LOST: 14 (6.4 kg)

TOTAL INCHES LOST: 19¼ (48.9 cm)

When I was young, my best friend and I were called Fat and Skinny. She was the fat one and I was the skinny one. We'd sit on the front porch and I would eat a whole bag of Doritos, a whole bag of Oreos and a diet cola. I could eat anything I wanted, and I never exercised. I never watched my weight because I never had to.

When I was pregnant with my first baby, I actually put on 6 stone 1 pound (38 kilograms) and then lost it all. During my second pregnancy, I put on about the same and I lost almost all of it except for maybe 5 pounds (2¼ kilograms). I probably weighed about 7 stone 12 pounds (50 kilograms). I stayed there for years and years. Then it started to creep up, and when I was 35, I weighed about 8 stone 3 pounds (52 kilograms). I stayed there until about the age of 42. Then I had a hysterectomy, so I went through the menopause, and I piled on about 1½ stone (9.6 kilograms) overnight. I started to exercise – I would run and work out, and I still ended up putting on weight.

Over the years, I've had several trainers and nutritionists. My first trainer got me to drink a lot of shakes. When you're drinking shakes and eating maybe one meal, you're going to lose the weight. I lost about 1½ stone (9.6 kilograms), and of course, I put it right back on. Then I went to another nutritionist, and I lost weight with her, too. But she limited me from having a lot of foods that I enjoy. The Skinny Chicks programme is very different from any of the other things I've tried. All women think we'll lose weight eating salads. Obviously, it's not true because most of the people who are eating salads are not thin. But they keep ordering salads.

I love eating all the foods we're allowed to eat. I didn't eat a lot of carbs before. I would only have them once in a while. Now I can have a carb at every meal, and I'm losing weight!

Losing weight makes me feel like myself again. Some people said I didn't need to lose weight. But it's not about what anybody else thinks; it's about what you *feel*. I felt horrible and I didn't want to go out or meet anybody because when you don't feel good about yourself, you're not going to feel good about anything.

It's really hard when you're going through the menopause, and just getting older in general, to lose weight and then keep it off. But this is working. The programme has definitely taught me a lot about nutrition and what happens to your body if you don't eat properly and you eat a lot of sugar, or if you eat only carbs or only protein, which is what I was doing. What a change this programme has made in my life. I plan to eat this way for ever.

getting to body fat). For that reason, if you *must* have a latte, mocha or macchiato, order them with skimmed milk, order the smallest size and drink them only along with a meal. Again, keep track of the total nutrient amounts and balances.

If You're Boozin', You Aren't Losin'

Let's face it. We all love to party after a hard day at the office, to celebrate a special occasion or just as a release of the tensions of everyday life. And for many of us, it's just not a party if there is no alcohol. However, if you really want to lose weight, you should bone up on your alcohol facts.

Drinking alcohol makes it much harder to lose body fat.

The liver normally prefers to break down proteins, carbs and most importantly fatty acids, but when pushy alcohol is present, all the nice little nutrients have to go to the end of the queue. Alcohol also permanently changes the structure of liver cells, which impairs the liver's ability to metabolize fats. So alcohol generally slows down weight loss. And of course, when you are tipsy or drunk, you are more likely to grab whatever you see and eat it. That doesn't help us fit into our little red dresses, now does it?

If you are truly going to lose weight, you must avoid all forms of alcohol as much as possible. Regardless of alcohol's 'benefits', it still slows down the metabolism of fatty acids within the liver and makes it more difficult to lose weight. While you're trying to lose weight, definitely avoid mixed drinks and spirits. Sorry! No more martinis, raspberry mojitos or margaritas. They are extremely high in calories.

So what is my advice? I say go out and buy yourself the most expensive bottle of red wine you can afford. Then, when you want to enjoy some, pour yourself a half-glass and enjoy it like it is the finest drink on Earth. You know you would rather have a quarter-glass of Chateau d'Yquem than a whole bottle of cheap plonk, and when it is that expensive, you definitely won't drink too much. Red wine contains antioxidants and resveratrol – a compound that has been observed to have an anti-clotting effect in the blood (believed to reduce the risk of heart

The Real Skinny on Beer Bellies

Some people believe that beer causes beer bellies because of the maltose (sugar) content in beer. The logic is that wine won't make you fat, but beer will because it is made of maltose. That would be correct if only it were that simple. Maltose is very high on the GI list – but beer is not pure maltose. Most beers contain only trace amounts of maltose since it is mostly fermented into alcohol. It's calories that cause beer bellies. Plenty of men who have never had a drop of beer have beer bellies, and indeed the term *beer belly* itself is a misnomer.

attacks and stroke). A small glass (about 60 millilitres/2 fluid ounces) has about 40 calories and will not slow down your weight loss. A standard-size serving of wine is about 150 millilitres (¼ pint), and some wine glasses hold much more than that – so it pays to measure the amount of wine you're drinking.

Here are some examples for you. These calorie counts are approximate, as every bartender has his or her own recipe and the calories vary according to ingredients and portions. But to give you a general idea:

COCKTAIL	CALORIES
Long Island Iced Tea	780
Frozen margarita	740
Margarita	490
Piña colada	460
Mai tai	350
Sangria	310
Martini	160–175
Mojito	150–220

PART III

SKINNY CHICKS

PUT IT ALL

TOGETHER

CHAPTER 11

Skinny Chicks Meal Plans

Now that you have the lowdown on why it's important to keep your blood sugar at a steady level and how the mighty PC Combo is the key to success, it's time to put all this great newfound knowledge into action. That's where my meal plans come in, and you'll find a week's worth of kick-start meals and 2 weeks of everyday meals in the pages that follow to get you up and running.

But don't stop there. The Skinny Chicks programme is designed to help you drop weight – serious amounts of weight – whether or not you incorporate exercise into your routine. But for optimal results and even greater, faster weight loss, I always recommend that my clients incorporate physical activity into their programmes as well as nutritional supplements. This section will give you guidelines for beginner, inter-mediate and advanced workouts to complement your meal plans as well as recommendations for safeguarding your health and well-being with dietary supplements.

If you're not currently exercising, I recommend you start with the beginner workout described on page 181 when you begin the kick-start programme. Once you gain strength and endurance, you can graduate to one of the more advanced workouts. If you already work out on a regular basis, start with the intermediate or advanced workouts.

About the Meal Plans

Kick-start meals have approximately the same calorie value as the everyday meals, but are comprised of foods (particularly carbs) in their most natural, minimally processed states. You will see that only unprocessed foods are called for; no bread, pasta, cereals or biscuits. You'll still be eating a healthy balance of carbs and proteins, but the carbs are whole grains, fruits and vegetables. I also recommend that you avoid restaurants and alcohol during this period. After 1 week, you can reintroduce some of the foods you've eliminated and enjoy an occasional meal out or a glass of wine.

While I have provided recipes for 1 full week of kick-start meals and 2 weeks' worth of everyday Skinny Chicks meals, I recognize that not everyone has time to cook even once or twice, much less four times every day. If that's true for you, don't worry! Many of these meals are choices you can find readily on restaurant menus or that you can replace with a frozen or ready-made meal (just be sure to chose one that has the proper ratio of carbs to protein; see page 162 for an example).

And if you really don't have time to cook at all, just choose a combination of foods from the kick-start or everyday food lists from the Appendix on page 275, keeping the total calories at or below 400 and again maintaining the proper ratio of carbs to protein.

Lastly, remember that all of these recipes, as well as those starting on page 235, can be used interchangeably. In that section you'll find all the recipes referred to in the kick-start and the everyday weight-loss plan, plus additional recipes that adhere to the Skinny Chicks guidelines to be used as the cornerstones of your own meal plans as you work toward meeting your individual weight-loss goal. As you've seen from the testimonials throughout this book, you can achieve remarkable results in just 10 weeks. Best of all, it's a way of eating you can really stick with. I should know; I've been doing it for 10 years and have enjoyed every minute of it.

The Skinny Chicks Kick-Start 7-Day Plan

Why a kick-start plan? The best way to start real-life weight loss is to clear out your internal system so that your body can begin to release stored body fat. When your body is loaded with toxins, it responds by retaining water in an effort to dilute water-soluble toxins. Your body also retains fat in an effort to dilute fat-soluble toxins. Until you clear your body of these toxins, it will work overtime to store water and fat to protect itself and dilute these toxins. In addition to clearing out toxins, the kick-start pro- gramme will help to stabilize blood sugar levels within the first few days. This is not a carbohydrate-restrictive programme; rather, you will be eating a PC Combo at every meal. However, the carbohydrate choices are all natu- ral, non-processed fresh fruits, vegetables and whole grains. **Please note: The kick-start plan is a strict nutrition programme and is only intended for short-term use.**

Benefits of the Kick-Start

1. You will drop 2 to 7 pounds (900 grams to 3.2 kilograms) or more of water, toxins and possibly body fat within 7 days.

2. As you lose weight, your body releases toxins from fat cells into the bloodstream, which can be harmful. Detoxification can help bind up these harmful toxins and move them out of the body safely.

3. If you have a large amount of body fat to lose and you hit a plateau at any point on the Skinny Chicks programme, it could be a result of too many toxins in your bloodstream. Coming back to the kick-start will probably break the plateau and get your fat burning going again.

Kick-Start Guidelines

- Eat a PC Combo every 4 hours.
- You can eat any meal at any time, i.e. breakfast for lunch. Make it your own and keep it simple for your lifestyle.

- Choose a lean protein and a fresh organic fruit or vegetable as your carbohydrate for each meal. You can cook vegetables; however, fresh and raw fruits and vegetables will yield the quickest weight loss on this programme. If you buy non-organic produce, soak and wash the produce with a 'veggie wash' to remove harmful chemicals, waxes and soil. Or use a bath of sea salt, a little vinegar and warm water.

- Nutrition facts for each meal are listed within the meal plans. To personalize your portions, use your palm as a guide for your protein portion and your fist with your opposite hand wrapped around it for your carbohydrate portion. You can cut your portions in half to substitute two snacks for a meal at any time.

- Choose a healthy fat such as extra virgin olive oil to cook with or to add flavour to your meal. Fat portions are approximately the size of a shot glass for nuts and half a shot glass for oils.

- Drink at least 10 glasses of water each day. Add a squirt of fresh lemon juice for added flavour and internal cleansing.

- Each day, drink at least 2 cups of cleansing tea that contains one of the following ingredients: dandelion and/or lemongrass.

- Consume no more than 120 milligrams of caffeine (the equivalent of 1 cup of coffee or 3 cups of green tea) per day.

- Avoid alcoholic beverages, desserts, preservatives and dining out as much as possible.

- Consume a minimum of three or four servings of fresh or frozen organically grown fruits and vegetables per day. See opposite for pointers on washing fruits and veggies.

- If you have access to a sauna and if you are not pregnant, sit in the sauna for 10 minutes each day. Toxins leave the body more readily when your core body temperature is elevated. This also promotes the release of human growth hormone, which is known to enhance youthfulness and foster better skin.

- Begin taking supplements: omega-3 fatty acids, a B-complex and a multivitamin. These will help speed up your detox, especially the B-complex.

- Repeat this plan for 1 to 4 weeks. Remember, you are free to mix and match all meals or repeat meals if need be. You can also mix and match the proteins, carbs and fats among the meals.

As you will see, I have separated the nutrients out for you. That way you can learn which foods are rich in protein, carbs and fat. The idea is to understand the predominant nutrient of each food you eat. Once you learn this, it becomes easy. Read through this meal plan carefully – learning the nutrients you get from foods is a cornerstone of your success.

There's also a box for 'free foods' – foods so low in calories and sugar that it is unnecessary to count their calories. 'Free foods' will not affect blood sugar levels, so enjoy! You can also find lists of my favourite proteins, carbs, fats and free foods in the Appendix, starting on page 275.

Variety is the spice of life, and in nutrition, variety is also healthy. But if you only find two or three meals that work for you, for the sake of simplicity, feel free to eat mostly those during your weight loss period (and be sure to take the supplements I recommend in Chapter 12).

Day 1

BREAKFAST

Pomegranate Blueberry Greek Yogurt

Combine all ingredients into a medium bowl and enjoy with a cup of warm cleansing tea (see page 120).

Nutrition facts: 320 calories, 27 g protein, 45 g carbohydrates, 9 g fat

PROTEIN POWERED	230 g (8 oz) 0% fat-free plain Greek yogurt
CARBOHYDRATE CONCENTRATED	seeds from ½ medium pomegranate, 30 g (1 oz) blueberries, 1 tbsp agave nectar
FAT FRIENDLY	1 tbsp crushed walnuts
FREE FOODS	Water, tea, coffee

CHRISTINE'S NUTRITION NUGGETS Pomegranates and blueberries are loaded with antioxidants that help reduce the risk of cancer and heart disease. They also enhance the production of glutathione, one of the most potent antioxidants in the body. Glutathione improves liver function and detoxification.

LUNCH

Grilled Salmon or Turkey Steak on a Bed of Rocket with Lemon

Serve the grilled salmon or turkey steak on a bed of rocket drizzled with extra virgin olive oil mixed with lemon juice, a dab of Dijon mustard and finely chopped garlic, with a serving of wild rice and a peach.

Nutrition facts: 363 calories, 28 g protein, 48 g carbohydrates, 8 g fat

PROTEIN POWERED	90-g (3-oz) (uncooked weight) salmon or turkey steak
CARBOHYDRATE CONCENTRATED	135 g (4¾ oz) cooked wild rice 1 peach
FAT FRIENDLY	1tsp extra virgin olive oil, omega-3s in the salmon
FREE FOODS	75 g (2½ oz) rocket Dab of Dijon mustard, lemon juice, and ½ tsp finely chopped garlic Water, tea

MID-AFTERNOON

High-Fibre, Low-Fat Protein Bar and Fruit

Grab and go!

Nutrition facts: 375 calories, 30 g protein, 40 g carbohydrates, 10 g fat

PROTEIN POWERED	1 high-fibre, low-fat protein bar (such as Labrada Lean Body Gold Bar)
CARBOHYDRATE CONCENTRATED	1 nectarine
FAT FRIENDLY	None; the fat in this meal comes in the protein bar.
FREE FOODS	Water, tea

DINNER

Oven-Roasted Chicken Breast, Rice or Quinoa, Carrots and Courgettes

Pair oven-roasted chicken breast (prepared at home or shop-bought) with brown rice or quinoa, steamed courgettes and carrots. Munch on frozen grapes for a sweet ending.

Nutrition facts: 381 calories, 27 g protein, 55 g carbohydrates, 7 g fat

PROTEIN POWERED	90 g (3 oz) oven-roasted skinless chicken breast
CARBOHYDRATE CONCENTRATED	100 g (3½ oz) cooked brown rice or quinoa 115 g (4 oz) steamed carrots 90 g (3 oz) frozen grapes
FAT FRIENDLY	1tsp extra virgin olive oil
FREE FOODS	Your choice of herbs and spices 115 g (4 oz) steamed courgettes Water, tea

DAY 2
BREAKFAST

Blueberry Blinis

Follow the recipe on page 238. Enjoy with a cup of cleansing tea (see page 120), plain or sweetened with a small drop of agave nectar.

Nutrition facts: 391 calories, 28 g protein, 56 g carbohydrates, 6 g fat

PROTEIN POWERED	Cottage cheese, cream cheese, egg whites
CARBOHYDRATE CONCENTRATED	Blueberry conserve, crepes, blueberries
FAT FRIENDLY	Cooking spray
FREE FOODS	Lemon juice

LUNCH

Baked Yam Stuffed with Peanut Butter, Cottage Cheese and Cinnamon

Wash and dry yam, then wrap with clingfilm and microwave 5–6 min. Remove clingfilm and slice yam lengthwise. Spread with peanut butter. Add cottage cheese, sprinkled with cinnamon and a drizzle of agave nectar.

Nutrition facts: 358 calories, 23 g protein, 46 g carbohydrates, 11 g fat

PROTEIN POWERED	170 g (6 z) low-fat cottage cheese
CARBOHYDRATE CONCENTRATED	Small yam (approx 115–145 g/4–5 oz) 1 tsp agave nectar
FAT FRIENDLY	1 tbsp natural peanut butter
FREE FOODS	Cinnamon Water, tea

MID-AFTERNOON

Hard-Boiled Eggs, Yogurt and Fruit

Mix sliced bananas with yogurt. Enjoy with eggs on the side.

Nutrition facts: 355 calories, 20 g protein, 48 g carbohydrates, 10 g fat

PROTEIN POWERED	2 hard-boiled omega-3 eggs
CARBOHYDRATE CONCENTRATED	170-g (6-oz) pot fat-free flavoured yogurt 1 small banana, sliced
FAT FRIENDLY	There are 10 grams of fat in the eggs. Thus, no additional fat is needed.
FREE FOODS	Water, tea

DINNER

Coconut Curry Sea Bass over Red Lentils

See recipe on page 256.

Nutrition facts: 344 calories, 25 g protein, 42 g carbohydrates, 9 g fat

PROTEIN POWERED	Sea bass
CARBOHYDRATE CONCENTRATED	Red lentils
FAT FRIENDLY	Extra virgin olive oil cooking spray Light coconut milk Unsweetened dessicated coconut
FREE FOODS	Red onion Coriander Finely chopped garlic Water, tea

CHRISTINE'S NUTRITION NUGGETS According to a 2007 US study, increased protein intake improved satiety at meals. What's more, protein provides important amino acids needed by the liver for detoxification, such as methionine and cysteine.

DAY 3
BREAKFAST

Wild Berry Parfait

Mix cottage cheese, strawberries, blueberries and berry yogurt; sprinkle with flaxseed or walnuts. Serve with a cup of cleansing tea (see page 120), plain or sweetened with a small drop of agave nectar.

Nutrition facts: 317 calories, 22 g protein, 45 g carbohydrates, 7 g fat

PROTEIN POWERED	170 g (6 oz) low-fat cottage cheese
CARBOHYDRATE CONCENTRATED	60 g (2 oz) each of strawberries and blueberries One 170-g (6-oz) container berry-flavoured low-fat yogurt
FAT FRIENDLY	2 tbsp ground flaxseed (linseed) or 1 tbsp crushed walnuts
FREE FOODS	Water, tea, coffee

LUNCH

Egg White Salad in Lettuce Cups and Fruit Salad

In a medium bowl, combine eggs, mayo, spring onions, celery, vinegar and salt and pepper to taste. Spoon egg salad into lettuce cups. Serve with mixed organic fruits.

Nutrition facts: 333 calories, 20 g protein, 44 g carbohydrates, 11 g fat

PROTEIN POWERED	5 hard-boiled egg whites, chopped
CARBOHYDRATE CONCENTRATED	½ fresh mango, sliced 115 g (4 oz) pineapple
FAT FRIENDLY	2 tbsp light mayo
FREE FOODS	1 tbsp finely chopped spring onions 1 tbsp diced celery 1 tsp cider vinegar Salt and ground black pepper Water, tea

MID-AFTERNOON

Citrus-y Greek Yogurt

Mix yogurt, sliced orange segments and walnuts in a medium bowl. Garnish with fresh mint leaf.

Nutrition facts: 332 calories, 28 g protein, 47 g carbohydrates, 5 g fat

PROTEIN POWERED	230 g (8 oz) 0% fat-free plain Greek yogurt
CARBOHYDRATE CONCENTRATED	1 large orange 1 tbsp agave nectar
FAT FRIENDLY	2 tbsp ground flaxseed (linseed) or 1 tbsp crushed nuts
FREE FOODS	Mint leaf Water, tea

DINNER

Herb-Crusted Salmon with Baby Potatoes and Artichokes

Steam artichoke over low heat for 30–40 minutes. Preheat oven to 180°C/350°F/gas 4. Line a baking tray with foil and spray with olive oil. Wash salmon, pat dry, and spread garlic, rosemary, salt and pepper over top. Bake for 10–15 min, depending on thickness. Serve with artichoke, steamed spinach and boiled potatoes.

Nutrition facts: 371 calories, 28 g protein, 52 g carbohydrates, 8 g fat

PROTEIN POWERED	90 g (3 oz) salmon
CARBOHYDRATE CONCENTRATED	170 g (6 oz) red potatoes 1 medium steamed artichoke
FAT FRIENDLY	Extra virgin olive oil cooking spray
FREE FOODS	30g (1 oz) spinach 1 tbsp finely chopped garlic 1 tbsp chopped rosemary Salt and ground black pepper Water, tea

CHRISTINE'S NUTRITION NUGGETS Artichokes have active compounds called caffeoylquinic acids or cynarin that prevent the build-up of fat and toxins in the liver. These compounds also act as a gentle laxative by increasing bile secretion.

DAY 4
BREAKFAST

Spinach and Feta Scramble (At Home or Dining Out)

To make at home, wilt spinach in a pan coated with olive oil cooking spray, add egg whites and scramble until cooked. Add feta, basil and tomato. For potatoes, wash, slice, sprinkle with salt and pepper to taste. Place in a glass bowl and cover with clingfilm. Microwave 2½ min. Enjoy a cup of cleansing tea (see page 120) plain or sweetened with a small drop of agave nectar and a small shot glass of pomegranate juice. If ordering at a restaurant, omit the cheese.

Nutrition facts: 319 calories, 23 g protein, 46 g carbohydrates, 5 g fat

PROTEIN POWERED	4 egg whites 2 tbsp low-fat feta cheese
CARBOHYDRATE CONCENTRATED	4 tbsp pomegranate juice 2 small baby potatoes
FAT FRIENDLY	Extra virgin olive oil cooking spray
FREE FOODS	15 g (½ oz) spinach leaves 1 basil leaf Tomato, chopped Salt and ground black pepper Water, tea, coffee

LUNCH

Tuna-Stuffed Celery Sticks with Fruit

In a medium bowl, combine tuna, egg, black olives, mayo, mustard, vinegar and onion. Season with salt and pepper to taste. Stuff tuna salad into celery sticks and enjoy with a fresh peach and pomegranate juice.

Nutrition facts: 340 calories, 22 g protein, 42 g carbohydrates, 10 g fat

PROTEIN POWERED	60 g (2 oz) light tuna chunks 1 hard-boiled egg, chopped
CARBOHYDRATE CONCENTRATED	Peach 120 ml (4 fl oz) pomegranate juice
FAT FRIENDLY	1 tbsp chopped black olives 1 tbsp light mayo
FREE FOODS	4 sticks celery 1 tsp chopped onion 1 tsp red wine vinegar 1 tsp Dijon mustard Salt and ground black pepper Water, tea

MID-AFTERNOON

Pumpkin Pie Cottage Cheese

Combine all ingredients in a medium bowl. Mix well. Sprinkle with cinnamon and enjoy.

Nutrition facts: 333 calories, 23 g protein, 49 g carbohydrates, 8 g fat

PROTEIN POWERED	170 g (6 oz) low-fat cottage cheese
CARBOHYDRATE CONCENTRATED	4 tbsp puréed pumpkin 2 tbsp raisins 2 tbsp agave nectar
FAT FRIENDLY	2 tbsp ground flaxseed (linseed)
FREE FOODS	Cinnamon Water, tea

CHRISTINE'S NUTRITION NUGGETS The insoluble fibre in ground flaxseed (linseed) acts as a natural laxative and increases regularity and elimination of toxins.

DINNER

Grilled White Fish with Quinoa or Brown Rice and Asparagus

Preheat grill to medium. Spray fish with olive oil spray, then rub with herbs and spices. Spray asparagus with olive oil spray and sprinkle with herbs and spices. Grill fish and asparagus until fish flakes easily with a fork. Serve with quinoa or brown rice. Finish with agave nectar-sweetened raspberries for dessert.

Nutrition facts: 380 calories, 26 g protein, 52 g carbohydrates, 8 g fat

PROTEIN POWERED	100 g (3½ oz) of white fish (any variety)
CARBOHYDRATE CONCENTRATED	135 g (4¾ oz) cooked quinoa or brown rice 60 g (2 oz) raspberries 1 tsp agave nectar
FAT FRIENDLY	Extra virgin olive oil cooking spray
FREE FOODS	Your favourite herbs and spices Asparagus spears (add salt and pepper to taste) Water, tea

DAY 5
BREAKFAST

Blueberry Peach Smoothie

Combine blueberries, peaches, protein powder, ice cubes, water and almond butter in a blender. Blend until thick and smooth. Enjoy with a cup of cleansing tea (see page 120), plain or sweetened with a small drop of agave nectar.

Nutrition facts: 377 calories, 26 g protein, 54 g carbohydrates, 10 g fat

PROTEIN POWERED	1 scoop vanilla-flavoured protein powder
CARBOHYDRATE CONCENTRATED	125 g (4½ oz) blueberries 125 g (4½ oz) peaches, sliced
FAT FRIENDLY	1 tbsp natural almond butter or 2 tsp flaxseed (linseed) oil
FREE FOODS	8 ice cubes 240–480 ml (8–16 fl oz) water Tea, coffee

 CHRISTINE'S NUTRITION NUGGETS All fruit is naturally low in fat, sodium and calories. Blueberries contain phytochemicals called anthocyanidins and proanthocyanins, which may play a role in preserving memory.

LUNCH

BBQ Chicken Breast, Corn on the Cob and Melon

BBQ the chicken however you like, prepare corn in boiling water or on grill, add salt to taste. Enjoy with a side of cantaloupe.

Nutrition facts: 393 calories, 27 g protein, 50 g carbohydrates, 12 g fat

PROTEIN POWERED	90 g (3 oz) BBQ skinless chicken breast
CARBOHYDRATE CONCENTRATED	½ cob of corn 2 cantaloupe wedges
FAT FRIENDLY	1 tsp extra virgin olive oil (brush onto chicken before grilling)
FREE FOODS	1 tbsp BBQ sauce Water, tea

MID-AFTERNOON

Turkey and Cheese Roll-Up

Wrap deli slices around cheese sticks and dip into Dijon mustard. Enjoy with grapefruit and sweet cherries.

Nutrition facts: 359 calories, 24 g protein, 58 g carbohydrates, 10 g fat

PROTEIN POWERED	2 sticks light cheese strings 2 slices deli turkey
CARBOHYDRATE CONCENTRATED	1 large grapefruit 90 g (3 oz) fresh cherries
FAT FRIENDLY	No need to add fat because there is fat in the string cheese.
FREE FOODS	Dijon mustard Water, tea

DINNER

Coriander Lime Sea Bass

See recipe on page 257, exchanging the couscous for brown rice.

Nutrition facts per serving: 350 calories, 22 g protein, 49 g carbohydrates, 10 g fat

PROTEIN POWERED	Sea bass
CARBOHYDRATE CONCENTRATED	Brown rice
FAT FRIENDLY	Extra virgin olive oil
FREE FOODS	Lime juice, coriander, ginger Water, tea

DAY 6
BREAKFAST

Veggie Delight Scramble

Wash potatoes and wrap in clingfilm. Microwave 4 min. In a medium frying pan coated with olive oil cooking spray, sautée onions, mushrooms and spinach 2 min over medium heat. Add egg whites and scramble until mostly cooked. Add chopped tomato and Cheddar and season with salt and pepper to taste. Serve with potatoes. Enjoy with a cup of of cleansing tea (see page 120), plain or sweetened with a small drop of agave nectar.

Nutrition facts: 327 calories, 25 g protein, 46 g carbohydrates, 5 g fat

PROTEIN POWERED	4 egg whites 2 tbsp low-fat Cheddar
CARBOHYDRATE CONCENTRATED	2 baby potatoes 340 g (12 oz) cubed watermelon
FAT FRIENDLY	Extra virgin olive oil cooking spray
FREE FOODS	1 tbsp chopped onion 15 g (½ oz) sliced mushrooms 15 g (½ oz) spinach 1 tbsp chopped tomato Salt and ground black pepper Water, tea, coffee

DINING OUT LUNCH

Sushi, Brown Rice and Steamed Veggies

Order at your favourite sushi hot spot!

Nutrition facts: 326 calories, 22 g protein, 44 g carbohydrates, 4 g fat

PROTEIN POWERED	2 pieces salmon roll 2 pieces tuna roll* 2 pieces yellowtail roll *If pregnant, swap tuna for salmon.
CARBOHYDRATE CONCENTRATED	Sushi is wrapped in rice, thus no need to add any other carbs to this meal.
FAT FRIENDLY	⅕ avocado, diced (rolled into sushi)
FREE FOODS	Less-salt soy sauce, wasabi 230 g (8 oz) steamed veggies Water, tea

MID-AFTERNOON

Deli Slices and Fruit

Combine mayo with honey mustard for dipping deli slices. Enjoy with 2 pieces of fresh summer fruit.

Nutrition facts: 318 calories, 17 g protein, 44 g carbohydrates, 8 g fat

PROTEIN POWERED	3 deli slices (turkey, ham or chicken)
CARBOHYDRATE CONCENTRATED	1 large peach 1 large nectarine
FAT FRIENDLY	1 tbsp light mayo
FREE FOODS	1 tbsp honey mustard Water, tea

DINNER

Cajun-Style Grilled Prawns and Brown Rice

See recipe on page 258.

Nutrition facts per serving: 410 calories, 28 g protein, 50 g carbohydrates, 11 g fat

PROTEIN POWERED	Grilled prawns
CARBOHYDRATE CONCENTRATED	Brown rice
FAT FRIENDLY	Extra virgin olive oil
FREE FOODS	Lemon juice Herbs and spices Water, tea

CHRISTINE'S NUTRITION NUGGETS Sushi is a healthy and delicious food; however, there are concerns of mercury in large predator fish such as bigeye and ahi tuna used for sushi. According to government data, these fish contain medium mercury levels (approximately 0.6 microgram per gram). The FDA says it's safe for women of childbearing age to consume two servings of tuna per week; however, I recommend avoiding tuna until you have finished breastfeeding.

DAY 7
BREAKFAST

Steel-Cut (Scotch) Oats with a Side Serving of Sweet Yogurt

Prepare porridge in water, according to the instructions on the packet. Top with fresh strawberry slices. Enjoy with a side serving of Greek yogurt drizzled with agave nectar and a cup of cleansing tea (see page 120), plain or sweetened with a small drop of agave nectar.

Nutrition facts: 347 calories, 25 g protein, 49 g carbohydrates, 6 g fat

PROTEIN POWERED	170 g (6 oz) 0% fat-free plain Greek yogurt
CARBOHYDRATE CONCENTRATED	100 g (3½ oz) cooked steel-cut (Scotch) oats (50 g/1¾ oz dry) 2 tsp agave nectar 30 g (1 oz) sliced strawberries
FAT FRIENDLY	2 tbsp ground flaxseed (linseed) or 1 tbsp slivered almonds
FREE FOODS	Water, tea, coffee

LUNCH

Roast Turkey Breast, Sweet Potato and Courgettes (At Home or Dining Out)

To make at home, roast turkey breast or reheat shop-bought. Wrap sweet potato in clingfilm and microwave 6–7 min. Remove clingfilm and slice lengthwise. Sprinkle with brown sugar. Steam courgettes with garlic salt and pepper.

Nutrition facts: 398 calories, 32 g protein, 56 g carbohydrates, 6 g fat

PROTEIN POWERED	90 g (3 oz) roasted skinless turkey breast
CARBOHYDRATE CONCENTRATED	1 medium (170-g/6-oz) sweet potato 1 tsp brown sugar
FAT FRIENDLY	Extra virgin olive oil cooking spray
FREE FOODS	Courgettes Garlic salt and ground black pepper Water, tea

MID-AFTERNOON

California Fruit Kebabs

See recipe on page 269. Sprinkle with nuts

Nutrition facts per serving: 313 calories, 27 g protein, 46 g carbohydrates, 4 g fat

PROTEIN POWERED	230 g (8 oz) 0% fat-free plain Greek yogurt
CARBOHYDRATE CONCENTRATED	Watermelon, honeydew melon, cantaloupe, strawberries, honey
FAT FRIENDLY	1 tbsp slivered almonds Cooking spray
FREE FOODS	Mint, water, tea

DINNER

Tex-Mex Chicken with Chipotle Sauce

See recipe on page 264.

Nutrition facts per serving: 380 calories, 24 g protein, 49 g carbohydrates, 11 g fat

PROTEIN POWERED	3 oz chicken breast
CARBOHYDRATE CONCENTRATED	Black beans, corn
FAT FRIENDLY	Avocado, olive oil Cooking spray
FREE FOODS	Coriander, lime, pepper, onion, tomatoes, jalapeño Water, tea

CHRISTINE'S NUTRITION NUGGETS Oats are a fantastic source of soluble fibre (which absorbs water; insoluble fibre does not). Soluble fibre helps to stabilize blood sugar levels, lowers cholesterol and curbs hunger. Soluble fibre also soaks up toxins in the intestines and moves them out of the body. Soluble fibre can also be found in apples, pears, grapefruits and artichokes.

The Skinny Chicks Everyday Weight Loss Plan

My general weight loss programme differs from the kick-start in that you will be allowed to enjoy wholemeal breads, crackers, cereal and pasta. Each meal is designed as a fat-burning PC Combo. Don't feel confused by all the options. Again, variety is healthy, but if you find two or three meals you love, feel free to eat those as often as you like during your weight loss period (and be sure to take the supplements I recommend in Chapter 12). If you have a large amount of body fat to lose and you hit a plateau at any point on the Skinny Chicks everyday programme, you may have too many toxins in your bloodstream. Returning to the kick-start plan for a week will help get your fat burning going again.

Most of the meals on this plan can be ordered at a restaurant; just remember to ask the chef to omit any cheeses, creams or cream sauces, guacamole, gravies or mayo. If they forget, you should remove or scrape off these items yourself. I have also included simple grab-and-go meals.

Everyday Meal Plan Guidelines

- Choose a lean protein, a healthy carbohydrate and fat for each meal.

- Eat a PC Combo every 4 hours, keeping the total calories for each below 400.

- Mix and match meals as you like. You can have breakfast for lunch and dinner for breakfast – whatever works best for your lifestyle.

- Remember to use your palm as a guide for your protein portion and your fist with your opposite hand wrapped around it for your carbohydrate portion. (Or you can use the measurements listed.)

- Recall that you are free to cut your portions in half to substitute two snacks for a meal at any time.

- Choose a healthy fat to cook with or to add flavour to your meal. Fat portions are approximately the size of a shot glass for nuts and half a shot glass for oils.

- Drink at least 10 glasses of water each day.

- Consume no more than 120 milligrams of caffeine (the equivalent of 1 cup of coffee or 3 cups of green tea) each day.

- Avoid alcoholic beverages, desserts, preservatives and dining out as much as possible.

- If you do choose to have an alcoholic beverage or dessert, be sure to reduce your meal portions.

- Consume **a minimum** of four to five servings of fresh or frozen organically grown fruits and vegetables per day. If you buy conventionally grown produce, soak and wash it with a 'veggie wash' to remove harmful chemicals. If you don't have veggie wash, you can use a solution of sea salt, vinegar and warm water. (Make this a habit in general, not only while you are on this programme!)

- Begin taking supplements: omega-3 fatty acids, B-complex and a multivitamin. These will help speed up your detox, especially the B-complex.

- Once weight loss goals are reached, continue to eat PC Combos to maintain weight loss results and overall good health, allowing yourself up to 450 calories per meal if you like.

As you will see, I have separated the nutrients out for you so you can learn the predominant nutrients of your foods. Once you learn this, it becomes easy. Remember that you can mix and match different kinds of proteins, carbs and fats if you like.

The 'free foods' – foods that are so low in calories and sugar that it is unnecessary to count their calories – will not affect blood sugar levels, so enjoy them. You can also find lists of my favourite proteins, carbs, fats and free foods in the Appendix.

DAY 1
BREAKFAST

Apple Maple Pecan Parfait

Combine all ingredients in a medium bowl and enjoy.

Nutrition facts: 384 calories, 26 g protein, 56 g carbohydrates, 8 g fat

PROTEIN POWERED	170 g (6 oz) low-fat cottage cheese
CARBOHYDRATE CONCENTRATED	One 170-g (6-oz) container low-fat vanilla yogurt 1 tbsp maple syrup ½ medium apple, diced
FAT FRIENDLY	2 tbsp crushed pecans
FREE FOODS	Water, tea, coffee

LUNCH

Turkey Sandwich, Baby Carrots and Fruit

Place turkey between bread slices, spread with avocado and Dijon mustard, and add your favourite 'free' veggies. Munch on baby carrots and apricots on the side. Enjoy!

Nutrition facts: 395 calories, 25 g protein, 51 g carbohydrates, 11 g fat

PROTEIN POWERED	3 slices smoked deli turkey
CARBOHYDRATE CONCENTRATED	2 slices wholemeal bread, toasted 2 small apricots 10 baby carrots
FAT FRIENDLY	⅕ medium Hass avocado
FREE FOODS	Dijon mustard Baby spinach leaves Tomato Red onion Water, tea

MID-AFTERNOON

Grilled Chicken Coriander Lime Wrap

Pile chicken and vegetables on a tortilla and top with fresh lime juice, coriander and salsa. Wrap and roll and enjoy with mango on the side.

Nutrition facts: 373 calories, 26 g protein, 47 g carbohydrates, 10 g fat

PROTEIN POWERED	90 g (3 oz) grilled skinless chicken breast
CARBOHYDRATE CONCENTRATED	1 medium wholewheat tortilla or pitta ½ medium fresh mango sliced
FAT FRIENDLY	Olive oil cooking spray ⅕ medium Hass avocado
FREE FOODS	Lime juice Chopped coriander Diced tomato Shredded lettuce Salsa Water, tea

DINNER

Fillet Steak with Mushroom Sauce and Herby Mashed Potatoes

See recipe on page 267, substituting fillet steak for the sirloin.

Nutrition facts per serving: 361 calories, 24 g protein, 50 g carbohydrates, 6 g fat

PROTEIN POWERED	Fillet steak
CARBOHYDRATE CONCENTRATED	Potatoes
FAT FRIENDLY	Extra virgin olive oil
FREE FOODS	Mushrooms Garlic, rosemary, thyme Chicken stock Water, tea

CHRISTINE'S NUTRITION NUGGETS Feel free to munch on 'free foods' – such as cucumber slices seasoned with rice vinegar, salt and freshly ground black pepper – between meals if you feel hungry. A nice warm cup of fruit-flavoured tea will also be enjoyable between meals. Tea contains an amino acid called L-theanine that has been proven to increase the activity of alpha brain waves, which increases awareness and calmness.

DAY 2
BREAKFAST

Berry Good Stuffed French Toast
See recipe on page 241.

Nutrition facts: 390 calories, 23 g protein, 53 g carbohydrates, 8 g fat

PROTEIN POWERED	Light cream cheese Egg whites
CARBOHYDRATE CONCENTRATED	Raspberry spread Fresh raspberries Wholemeal bread
FAT FRIENDLY	Cooking spray
FREE FOODS	Mint leaf Water, tea, coffee

LUNCH

Chicken Soft Taco (At Home or Dining Out)
Wrap chicken into warm tortilla with lettuce, tomato, onion and salsa. Enjoy black beans and rice on the side. If dining out, order two chicken soft tacos and request no cheese, no soured cream and no special sauces except for salsa.

Nutrition facts: 388 calories, 29 g protein, 56 g carbohydrates, 7 g fat

PROTEIN POWERED	90 g (3 oz) grilled skinless chicken breast
CARBOHYDRATE CONCENTRATED	One 15-cm (6-in) wholewheat tortilla 40 g (1¼ oz) black beans 40 g (1¼ oz) rice
FAT FRIENDLY	Extra virgin olive oil cooking spray
FREE FOODS	Shredded lettuce Tomato Onion Fresh salsa Water, tea

MID-AFTERNOON

Apple Cinnamon Cottage Cheese

Combine all ingredients in a medium bowl, and mix well. Enjoy!

Nutrition facts: 338 calories, 22 g protein, 47 g carbohydrates, 7 g fat

PROTEIN POWERED	170 g (6 oz) low-fat cottage cheese
CARBOHYDRATE CONCENTRATED	170 g (6 oz) unsweetened organic stewed apple
FAT FRIENDLY	1 pinch slivered almonds
FREE FOODS	Cinnamon Water, tea

DINNER

Christine's Pasta and Spicy Red Sauce

See recipe on page 249.

Nutrition facts per serving: 425 calories, 31 g protein, 59 g carbohydrates, 9 g fat

PROTEIN POWERED	115 g (4 oz) extra-lean turkey mince Parmesan cheese
CARBOHYDRATE CONCENTRATED	115 g (4 oz) cooked wholewheat pasta Tomato sauce
FAT FRIENDLY	Extra virgin olive oil
FREE FOODS	Onion Green pepper Garlic Chopped tomatoes Water, tea

CHRISTINE'S NUTRITION NUGGETS Tomatoes are loaded with lycopene, a powerful antioxidant that has been proven to reduce the risk of cardiovascular disease and prostate and gastrointestinal cancers. So load up on that red sauce!

DAY 3
BREAKFAST

Breakfast Bagel Sandwich
(At Home or Dining Out)

To make at home, see recipe on page 239.

Nutrition facts per serving: 369 calories, 27 g protein, 44 g carbohydrates, 9 g fat

PROTEIN POWERED	Canadian bacon Egg whites Light cream cheese
CARBOHYDRATE CONCENTRATED	Wholemeal bagel
FAT FRIENDLY	Cooking spray Omega-3 spread
FREE FOODS	Tomato

LUNCH

Cheese and Veggie Quesadilla

Coat a medium frying pan with cooking spray. Warm tortilla over medium heat until it begins to brown. Add grated cheese. Once cheese is melted, add your favourite free veggies and condiments and serve.

Nutrition facts: 346 calories, 24 g protein, 52 g carbohydrates, 5 g fat

PROTEIN POWERED	60 g (2 oz) low-fat grated Cheddar or light mozzarella cheese
CARBOHYDRATE CONCENTRATED	One 15-cm (6-in) wholewheat or corn tortilla 1 large watermelon wedge
FAT FRIENDLY	⅛ medium Hass avocado Extra virgin olive oil cooking spray
FREE FOODS	Tomato Onion Salsa 1 tbsp low-fat soured cream Water, tea

MID-AFTERNOON

Turkey Slice, Cherries and Trail Mix
Grab and go!

Nutrition facts: 334 calories, 20 g protein, 42 g carbohydrates, 13 g fat

PROTEIN POWERED	1 deli slice (turkey or chicken)
CARBOHYDRATE CONCENTRATED	30 g (1 oz) fresh cherries 115 g (4 oz) unsalted trail mix
FAT FRIENDLY	Nuts in the trail mix
FREE FOODS	Water, tea

DINNER

Wasabi Sesame Salmon with Brown Rice Noodles
See recipe on page 253.

Nutrition facts per serving: 400 calories, 25 g protein, 48 g carbohydrates,
12 g fat

PROTEIN POWERED	Salmon
CARBOHYDRATE CONCENTRATED	Brown rice spaghetti Carrots
FAT FRIENDLY	Light mayo Sesame seeds
FREE FOODS	Wasabi, soy sauce, chicken stock, chilli sauce Spring onions

CHRISTINE'S NUTRITION NUGGETS Salmon is packed with heart-healthy omega-3 fatty acids, which are known to lower blood pressure.

DAY 4
BREAKFAST

Peanut Butter Toast

Spread peanut butter on toast and place 60 g (2 oz) cottage cheese on each slice of toast. Sprinkle with cinnamon and enjoy with ½ banana on the side.

Nutrition facts: 359 calories, 23 g protein, 43 g carbohydrates, 11 g fat

PROTEIN POWERED	115 g (4 oz) low-fat cottage cheese
CARBOHYDRATE CONCENTRATED	2 slices wholemeal bread or 1 wholemeal English muffin ½ small banana
FAT FRIENDLY	1 tbsp natural peanut butter
FREE FOODS	Cinnamon Water, tea, coffee

LUNCH

Blue Cheese Chicken Burger (At Home or Dining Out)

Spread toasted bun with Dijon mustard and light mayo, then add chicken burger, blue cheese, lettuce, tomato and onion. Garnish with a pickle. Enjoy with a fresh wedge of watermelon. If dining out, omit the cheese; if fresh fruit is not available, replace with a small natural lemonade (not fizzy).

Nutrition facts: 412 calories, 30 g protein, 57 g carbohydrates, 9 g fat

PROTEIN POWERED	90 g (3 oz) grilled skinless chicken breast 1 tbsp reduced-fat blue cheese
CARBOHYDRATE CONCENTRATED	1 small wholemeal bap 1 large watermelon wedge, or 1 c cubed
FAT FRIENDLY	Extra virgin olive oil cooking spray (for grilling) 1 tbsp light mayo
FREE FOODS	Dijon mustard Lettuce Tomato Onion Pickle Water, tea

MID-AFTERNOON

Citrus-y Greek Yogurt

See recipe on page 127. Cut orange into segments and combine in a medium bowl with remaining ingredients. Garnish with fresh mint leaf and enjoy.

Nutrition facts: 332 calories, 28 g protein, 47 g carbohydrates, 5 g fat

CHRISTINE'S NUTRITION NUGGETS Low-fat dairy products contain higher amounts of protein, vitamin D and calcium, and less disease-causing saturated fat.

DINNER

Grilled Chicken Fajitas

See recipe on page 263 or order at your favourite Tex-Mex restaurant. A portion should be two 15-cm (6 in) tortillas filled with ingredients.

Nutrition facts per serving: 417 calories, 30 g protein, 56 g carbohydrates, 8 g fat

PROTEIN POWERED	Grilled skinless chicken breast
CARBOHYDRATE CONCENTRATED	Wholewheat or corn tortillas
FAT FRIENDLY	Extra virgin olive oil cooking spray
FREE FOODS	Pepper Onion Tomato Salsa Lime juice Low-fat soured cream Water, tea

DAY 5

BREAKFAST

Berry Delish Porridge

Prepare porridge in water according to the instructions on the packet. Add protein powder immediately after cooking. Top with berries, agave nectar and slivered almonds, and sprinkle with cinnamon.

Nutrition facts: 366 calories, 23 g protein, 56 g carbohydrates, 7 g fat

PROTEIN POWERED	½ scoop protein powder 120 ml (4 fl oz) nonfat milk or soy milk
CARBOHYDRATE CONCENTRATED	100 g (3½ oz) cooked porridge 60 g (2 oz) blueberries, fresh or frozen 60 g (2 oz) strawberries, fresh or frozen 2 tsp agave nectar
FAT FRIENDLY	1 tbsp slivered almonds
FREE FOODS	Cinnamon Water, tea, coffee

LUNCH

Greek Chicken Pitta with Cucumber and Mint

Spread hummus inside pitta. Stuff chicken, cucumber, onion, tomato and mint into pitta. Season with vinegar, salt and pepper, and drizzle lightly with extra virgin olive oil. Enjoy with fresh grapes.

Nutrition facts: 401 calories, 28 g protein, 54 g carbohydrates, 10 g fat

PROTEIN POWERED	75 g (2½ oz) grilled skinless chicken breast 1 tbsp low-fat feta cheese
CARBOHYDRATE CONCENTRATED	Wholemeal pitta 75 g (2½ oz) seedless grapes
FAT FRIENDLY	1 tbsp hummus 1 tsp extra virgin olive oil
FREE FOODS	Cucumber, red onion, tomato Fresh mint leaves Red wine vinegar Salt and freshly ground black pepper Water, tea

MID-AFTERNOON

Low-Fat Egg White Salad and Crispbreads

In a medium bowl, combine egg whites, mayo, bell pepper, onion, vinegar and salt to taste. Serve with crispbreads and fresh strawberries.

Nutrition facts: 403 calories, 26 g protein, 52 g carbohydrates, 10 g fat

PROTEIN POWERED	5 hard-boiled egg whites
CARBOHYDRATE CONCENTRATED	2 wholegrain crispbreads (like Dr Karg) 10 strawberries
FAT FRIENDLY	1 tbsp light mayo
FREE FOODS	1 tbsp chopped green pepper 1 tbsp chopped red onion I tsp cider vinegar Salt Water, tea

DINNER

Mediterranean Prawn Pasta

See recipe on page 251. Or order at a restaurant: ask for pasta with a stock-based sauce and grilled prawns. Eat half of the restaurant portion.

Nutrition facts per serving: 399 calories, 30 g protein, 48 g carbohydrates, 10 g fat

PROTEIN POWERED	Prawns
CARBOHYDRATE CONCENTRATED	Brown rice pasta
FAT FRIENDLY	Extra virgin olive oil
FREE FOODS	Tomatoes Spinach Garlic Lemon Basil Water, tea

CHRISTINE'S NUTRITION NUGGETS Garlic is loaded with allyl sulphides, which have been proven to reduce the risk of cancer in multiple research studies.

DAY 6
BREAKFAST

Onion and Tomato Egg White Scramble (At Home or Dining Out)

To make at home, coat a medium frying pan with cooking spray. Add sliced spring onion, salt and pepper and sautée on medium–low heat for 2 min. Add egg whites and scramble until almost cooked. Add diced tomato and low-fat cheese. Serve with 1 toasted English muffin spread lightly with peanut butter.

Nutrition facts: 325 calories, 23 g protein, 44 g carbohydrates, 6 g fat

PROTEIN POWERED	5 egg whites 30 g (1 oz) low-fat cheese
CARBOHYDRATE CONCENTRATED	½ wholemeal English muffin 240 ml (8 fl oz) orange juice
FAT FRIENDLY	Extra virgin olive oil cooking spray 1 tbsp natural peanut butter
FREE FOODS	Spring onions Tomato Salt and ground black pepper Water, tea, coffee

LUNCH

Veggie and Cheese Sandwich

Spread mashed avocado and light mayo on each slice of bread. Add your favourite 'free' vegetables and enjoy with fresh apricots or any small fruit.

Nutrition facts: 371 calories, 26 g protein, 47 g carbohydrates, 8 g fat

PROTEIN POWERED	3 small slices low-fat cheese
CARBOHYDRATE CONCENTRATED	2 slices wholemeal bread 1 tbsp grated carrots 3 small apricots
FAT FRIENDLY	1 tbsp mashed avocado 1 tbsp light mayo
FREE FOODS	Cucumber, alfalfa sprouts, spinach leaves, red onion, tomato Water, tea

MID-AFTERNOON

Grilled Salmon Steak with Rocket

Spread toasted burger bun with Dijon mustard and top with grilled salmon steak, rocket, tomato and onion. Garnish with gherkins. Enjoy with a delicious pomegranate.

Nutrition facts: 399 calories, 27 g protein, 55 g carbohydrates, 4 g fat

PROTEIN POWERED	90 g (3 oz) (uncooked weight) salmon
CARBOHYDRATE CONCENTRATED	1 small wholemeal bap 1 fresh medium pomegranate
FAT FRIENDLY	The salmon contains healthy fat.
FREE FOODS	Dijon mustard Rocket, tomato, red onion Gherkins Water, tea

 CHRISTINE'S NUTRITION NUGGETS Rocket is packed with vitamin A – about 10 percent of your recommended daily intake, or RDI, per cup. Vitamin A is beneficial in preventing night blindness, skin disorders and even acne.

DINNER

Christine's Enchiladas

See recipe on page 266. Allow two enchiladas and 65 g (2¼ oz) rice per serving.

Nutrition facts per serving: 372 calories, 28 g protein, 54 g carbohydrates, 7 g fat

PROTEIN POWERED	Turkey mince Low-fat Cheddar cheese
CARBOHYDRATE CONCENTRATED	Tortillas Rice
FAT FRIENDLY	Extra virgin olive oil
FREE FOODS	Coriander, onion, green chilli peppers, garlic, crushed chillies, spices, salsa, low-fat soured cream Water, tea

DAY 7
BREAKFAST

Blueberry Yogurt Parfait with Slivered Almonds

In a medium bowl, combine all ingredients and mix well. Enjoy!

Nutrition facts: 308 calories, 22 g protein, 46 g carbohydrates, 5 g fat

PROTEIN POWERED	115 g (4 oz) low-fat cottage cheese
CARBOHYDRATE CONCENTRATED	One 170-g (6-oz) container low-fat yogurt Handful blueberries
FAT FRIENDLY	1 tbsp slivered almonds
FREE FOODS	Water, tea, coffee

LUNCH

Grilled Chicken Sandwich (At Home or Dining Out)

Spread bap with Dijon mustard and mayo or avocado. Place chicken breast, spinach, onion and tomato in bap. Enjoy with an apple. If eating out, order a 12" chicken sandwich from Subway. Save half for mid-afternoon.

Nutrition facts: 395 calories, 25 g protein, 51 g carbohydrates, 11 g fat

PROTEIN POWERED	90 g (3 oz) grilled skinless chicken breast 1 small slice of low-fat cheese (optional)
CARBOHYDRATE CONCENTRATED	1 small wholemeal bap 1 medium apple
FAT FRIENDLY	Cooking spray 1 tbsp light mayo or mashed avocado
FREE FOODS	Dijon mustard Spinach leaves Red onion Tomato Water, tea

MID-AFTERNOON

Pumpkin Pie Cottage Cheese

See Kick-Start Day 4, on page 129.

Nutrition facts: 333 calories, 23 g protein, 49 g carbohydrates, 8 g fat

DINNER

Coriander Lime Sea Bass

See recipe on page 257. Serve raspberries with agave nectar for dessert.

Nutrition facts per serving: 350 calories, 22 g protein, 49 g carbohydrates, 10 g fat

PROTEIN POWERED	90 g (3 oz) sea bass
CARBOHYDRATE CONCENTRATED	180 g (6½ oz) couscous 2 tbsp raisins 60 g (2 oz)raspberries ½ tbsp agave nectar
FAT FRIENDLY	Extra virgin olive oil
FREE FOODS	Lime juice, coriander, ginger Water, tea

CHRISTINE'S NUTRITION NUGGETS Coriander contains an antibacterial compound that may prove to be a natural means for fighting *Salmonella*. Pumpkin has been shown to help manage hyperglycemia and hypertension.

DAY 8
BREAKFAST

Breakfast Bagel Sandwich
See recipe on page 240.

Nutrition facts per serving: 369 calories, 27 g protein, 44 g carbohydrates, 9 g fat

PROTEIN POWERED	Canadian bacon Liquid egg whites Light cream cheese
CARBOHYDRATE CONCENTRATED	Wholemeal bagel
FAT FRIENDLY	Cooking spray Omega-3 light spread
FREE FOODS	Tomato Water, tea, coffee

LUNCH

Baked Nacho Chips and Cheesy Salsa
In a medium bowl, combine cottage cheese, olives and 'free' veggies and mix well. Dip baked chips into cheesy salsa mixture and enjoy.

Nutrition facts: 357 calories, 23 g protein, 47 g carbohydrates, 9 g fat

PROTEIN POWERED	170 g (6 oz) low-fat, low-sodium cottage cheese
CARBOHYDRATE CONCENTRATED	25 baked tortilla chips
FAT FRIENDLY	9 black olives, diced
FREE FOODS	3 sliced spring onions 1 tbsp diced jalapeño chilli peppers ¼ red pepper, diced Salsa Water, tea

MID-AFTERNOON

Fruity Bagel Dippers

In a medium bowl, combine all ingredients except bagel and your drink, and mix well. Dip bagel into mix. Enjoy!

Nutrition facts: 380 calories, 25 g protein, 64 g carbohydrates, 4 g fat

PROTEIN POWERED	115 g (4 oz) low-fat cottage cheese
CARBOHYDRATE CONCENTRATED	One 170-g (6-oz) container low-fat yogurt Handful of blueberries 1 wholemeal bagel
FAT FRIENDLY	1 pinch slivered almonds
FREE FOODS	Water, tea

DINNER

Christine's Born-Again Lasagne

See recipe on page 252.

Nutrition facts per serving: 467 calories, 34 g protein, 61 g carbohydrates, 8 g fat

PROTEIN POWERED	Turkey mince Low-fat ricotta cheese Light Mozzarella cheese
CARBOHYDRATE CONCENTRATED	Wholewheat lasagne noodles Pasta sauce 1 slice wholemeal sourdough bread
FAT FRIENDLY	Extra virgin olive oil
FREE FOODS	Garlic Green pepper Mushrooms Spices Water, tea

CHRISTINE'S NUTRITION NUGGETS Avocado is packed with vitamin E, which is great for preventing the onset of cardiovascular disease. It's also packed with soluble fibre, which helps to stabilize blood sugar.

DAY 9
BREAKFAST

Cinnamon Raisin Oaty Muffins
See recipe on page 240.

Nutrition facts per serving: 365 calories, 25 g protein, 54 g carbohydrates, 9 g fat

PROTEIN POWERED	Egg whites Low-fat cottage cheese Protein powder
CARBOHYDRATE CONCENTRATED	Oats Raisins
FAT FRIENDLY	Cooking spray Omega-3 spread
FREE FOODS	Cinnamon Agave nectar

LUNCH

Sandwich and Baked Tortilla Chips (At Home or Dining Out)
To make at home, spread mustard and mayo on each slice of bread. Place turkey and favourite veggies into sandwich. Enjoy with 1 handful of baked tortilla chips and a pickled gherkin.

Nutrition facts: 434 calories, 27 g protein, 62 g carbohydrates, 10 g fat

PROTEIN POWERED	3 slices turkey breast
CARBOHYDRATE CONCENTRATED	10 baked tortilla chips (or 1 handful) 2 slices of wholemeal bread
FAT FRIENDLY	1 tbsp light mayo
FREE FOODS	Dijon mustard Onion Lettuce Tomato Pickled gherkin Water, tea

MID-AFTERNOON

High-Fibre, Low-Fat Protein Bar with Anjou Pear

Grab and go!

Nutrition facts: 400 calories, 30 g protein, 40 g carbohydrates, 8 g fat

PROTEIN POWERED	Low-fat, high-fibre protein bar (such as Labrada Lean Body Gold Bar)
CARBOHYDRATE CONCENTRATED	1 medium Anjou pear
FAT FRIENDLY	There is fat in the protein bar.
FREE FOODS	Water, tea

DINNER

Chicken Kebabs with Rice (At Home or Dining Out)

To make at home, see recipe on page 262 or order at any Greek restaurant. Omit the hummus as it's loaded with olive oil – a good fat, but too much will cause weight gain.

Nutrition facts: 377 calories, 22 g protein, 45 g carbohydrates, 12 g fat

PROTEIN POWERED	75 g (2½ oz) grilled skinless chicken breast
CARBOHYDRATE CONCENTRATED	65 g (2¼ oz) rice
FAT FRIENDLY	Extra virgin olive oil spray
FREE FOODS	Garlic Pepper Mushroom Tomato Water, tea

CHRISTINE'S NUTRITION NUGGETS Remember that you are free to cut your meal in half at any time and enjoy 'free' veggies between meals. Peppers are one of the three important veggies – broccoli, peppers and Brussels sprouts – that are a good source of vitamin C.

DAY 10
BREAKFAST

Apple Raisin Porridge

Prepare porridge according to the instructions on the packet. Add raisins, apples and cinnamon. Enjoy with a side serving of egg whites to keep blood sugar stable.

Nutrition facts: 349 calories, 22 g protein, 51 g carbohydrates, 7 g fat

PROTEIN POWERED	4 egg whites, hard-boiled or scrambled
CARBOHYDRATE CONCENTRATED	100 g (3½ oz) slow-cooked steel-cut (Scotch porridge) oats 2 tbsp raisins 60 g (2 oz) diced apple
FAT FRIENDLY	1 tbsp slivered almonds
FREE FOODS	Cinnamon Sweetener such as Splenda Water, tea, coffee

LUNCH

Low-Fat Tuna Sandwich

In a medium bowl, combine tuna, egg, black olives, mayo, Dijon mustard, relish, celery and onion. Season with salt and pepper to taste. Place mixture onto bread slices and top with cucumber, alfalfa sprouts and tomato. Enjoy with pomegranate juice.

Nutrition facts: 395 calories, 28 g protein, 45 g carbohydrates, 12 g fat

PROTEIN POWERED	60 g (2 oz) chunky light tuna* 1 hard-boiled egg, diced *If pregnant, use sliced chicken breast instead.
CARBOHYDRATE CONCENTRATED	2 slices wholemeal bread 60 ml (2 fl oz) pomegranate juice
FAT FRIENDLY	1 tbsp diced black olives 1 tbsp light mayo
FREE FOODS	1 tsp Dijon mustard 1 tsp gherkin relish Celery and onion, diced Salt and ground black pepper Cucumber, alfalfa sprouts, tomato Water, tea

MID-AFTERNOON

String Cheese and Fruit

Grab and go!

Nutrition facts: 306 calories, 20 g protein, 44 g carbohydrates, 8 g fat

PROTEIN POWERED	3 sticks light cheese strings
CARBOHYDRATE CONCENTRATED	150 g (5½ oz) red seedless grapes
FAT FRIENDLY	No need to add fat because there is fat in the string cheese.
FREE FOODS	Water, tea

DINNER

Smoked Salmon Bagel

Toast bagel and spread with cream cheese. Place salmon, olives and 'free' veggies on bagel and enjoy.

Nutrition facts: 392 calories, 32 g protein, 58 g carbohydrates, 5 g fat

PROTEIN POWERED	1 slice smoked salmon 2 tbsp light cream cheese
CARBOHYDRATE CONCENTRATED	Wholemeal bagel
FAT FRIENDLY	There is heart-healthy fat in the salmon.
FREE FOODS	Tomato Green onion Water, tea

CHRISTINE'S NUTRITION NUGGETS Eggs are an excellent source of biotin, a vitamin used in breaking down fat, protein and carbs.

DAY 11
BREAKFAST

Honey Nut Apple Crunch

In a medium bowl, mix all ingredients together and enjoy.

Nutrition facts: 367 calories, 27 g protein, 58 g carbohydrates, 5 g fat

PROTEIN POWERED	230 g (8 oz) 0% fat-free plain Greek yogurt
CARBOHYDRATE CONCENTRATED	1 large diced apple 1 tbsp honey or agave nectar
FAT FRIENDLY	1 tbsp crushed walnuts
FREE FOODS	Cinnamon Water, tea, coffee

LUNCH

Christine's Super Bowl Sunday Nachos

Place baked tortilla chips on a large, microwave-safe plate. Cover evenly with cheese and microwave 60 sec. Add remaining ingredients and enjoy.

Nutrition facts: 377 calories, 25 g protein, 47 g carbohydrates, 8 g fat

PROTEIN POWERED	75 g (2½ oz) low-fat Cheddar cheese, grated
CARBOHYDRATE CONCENTRATED	30 baked tortilla chips (or 3 handfuls)
FAT FRIENDLY	9 black olives, diced
FREE FOODS	¼ green pepper 3 sliced spring onions 1 tbsp diced jalapeño chilli peppers 1 medium tomato, diced Salsa Water, tea

MID-AFTERNOON

Healthy Pizza

Preheat oven to 190ºC/375ºF/gas 5. Spread 115 g (4 oz) tomato pasta sauce on each half of bagel. Add cheese, olives and your favourite 'free' veggies and place on a baking sheet covered with aluminium foil. Toast in oven for 10–15 min, or until desired doneness.

Nutrition facts: 390 calories, 28 g protein, 58 g carbohydrates, 6 g fat

PROTEIN POWERED	60 g (2 oz) grated mozzarella cheese
CARBOHYDRATE CONCENTRATED	1 toaster-size wholemeal bagel 230 g (8 oz) tomato pasta sauce
FAT FRIENDLY	5 black olives, sliced
FREE FOODS	Onion Mushrooms Green pepper Finely chopped garlic Water, tea

DINNER

Grilled Halibut with Quinoa and Asparagus

Preheat grill to medium heat. Brush fish with olive oil, then rub with your favourite spices. Brush asparagus spears with olive oil and sprinkle with your favourite spices. Place fish and asparagus on grill and cook until fish flakes easily. Serve with quinoa or brown rice. Finish with raspberries sweetened with agave nectar for dessert.

Nutrition facts: 360 calories, 28 g protein, 47 g carbohydrates, 9 g fat

PROTEIN POWERED	100 g (3½ oz) halibut, raw
CARBOHYDRATE CONCENTRATED	90 g (3 oz) cooked quinoa 90 g (3 oz) raspberries 2 tsp agave nectar
FAT FRIENDLY	1 tsp extra virgin olive oil
FREE FOODS	Herbs, spices Asparagus spears Water, tea

CHRISTINE'S NUTRITION NUGGETS Quinoa is a grain that is similar to rice, yet it offers more fibre and protein per serving. Best of all, quinoa also contains the nine essential amino acids.

DAY 12
BREAKFAST

Breakfast Bagel Sandwich
See recipe on page 239.

Nutrition facts per serving: 369 calories, 27 g protein, 44 g carbohydrates, 9 g fat

PROTEIN POWERED	Canadian bacon Liquid egg whites Light cream cheese
CARBOHYDRATE CONCENTRATED	Wholemeal bagel
FAT FRIENDLY	Cooking spray Omega-3 light spread
FREE FOODS	Tomato Salt and ground black pepper

LUNCH

Super-Fast Tuscan Polenta
Cut polenta into 1-cm (½-in)-thick slices. Using a spoon to partially hollow out the centres, spread polenta slices with tomato pasta sauce. Sprinkle with cheese and microwave 1–2 min. Top with chopped basil and enjoy!

Nutrition facts: 320 calories, 25 g protein, 50 g carbohydrates, 2 g fat

PROTEIN POWERED	60 g (2 oz) grated mozzarella cheese
CARBOHYDRATE CONCENTRATED	30 g (1 oz) ready-made polenta 115 g (4 oz) low-fat tomato pasta sauce
FAT FRIENDLY	Olive oil cooking spray
FREE FOODS	1 basil leaf Water, tea

MID-AFTERNOON

Deli Slices and Fruit

Combine mayo with honey mustard. Roll and dip slices into mixture. Enjoy with 2 pieces of summer fresh fruit.

Nutrition facts: 318 calories, 17 g protein, 44 g carbohydrates, 8 g fat

PROTEIN POWERED	3 deli slices (turkey, ham or chicken)
CARBOHYDRATE CONCENTRATED	1 large peach 1 large nectarine
FAT FRIENDLY	1 tbsp light mayo
FREE FOODS	1 tbsp honey mustard Water, tea

DINNER

Baked Turkey, Sweet Potato and Steamed Broccoli (At Home or Dining Out)

To make at home, roast a turkey breast or buy ready-prepared. Wrap sweet potato with clingfilm and microwave 6–7 min; remove clingfilm and slice down the middle. Sprinkle with brown sugar. Steam broccoli with garlic salt and pepper. Add a little lemon juice. Serve and enjoy.

Nutrition facts: 398 calories, 32 g protein, 56 g carbohydrates, 6 g fat

PROTEIN POWERED	90 g (3 oz) roasted skinless turkey breast
CARBOHYDRATE CONCENTRATED	1 medium (170-g/6-oz) sweet potato 1 tsp brown sugar
FAT FRIENDLY	Extra virgin olive oil spray
FREE FOODS	Broccoli Garlic salt and freshly ground black pepper Lemon juice Water, tea

CHRISTINE'S NUTRITION NUGGETS The fatty acids in fish oil and olive oil not only help with the prevention of heart disease but also have an anti-inflammatory effect.

DAY 13
BREAKFAST

Chocolate Peanut Butter Smoothie

Place all ingredients into a blend and mix until consistency is smooth and creamy. Enjoy!

Nutrition facts: 335 calories, 25 g protein, 44 g carbohydrates, 9 g fat

PROTEIN POWERED	1 scoop chocolate-flavoured protein powder
CARBOHYDRATE CONCENTRATED	2 small frozen bananas
FAT FRIENDLY	1 tbsp natural peanut butter
FREE FOODS	10 ice cubes 240–480 ml (8–16 fl oz) water Tea, coffee

LUNCH

Frozen Meal (Any brand that has approximately 1 part protein to 2 parts carbs)

Find any frozen meal that is high in protein and low in fat such as Chicken Florentine by Lean Cuisine Healthy Portions. If the carbs are too low, you can add a small piece of fruit to your meal. Then just zap and go!

PROTEIN POWERED	Chicken
CARBOHYDRATE CONCENTRATED	Carrots Pasta
FAT FRIENDLY	Most frozen meals contain fat. If not, have a serving of nuts on the side.
FREE FOODS	Water, tea

MID-AFTERNOON

Greek Yogurt with Honey and Walnuts

Combine ingredients in a medium bowl and enjoy.

Nutrition facts: 363 calories, 29 g protein, 52 g carbohydrates, 6 g fat

PROTEIN POWERED	230 g (8 oz) 0% fat-free plain Greek yogurt
CARBOHYDRATE CONCENTRATED	45 g (1½ oz) low-fat granola 30 g (1 oz) blueberries 1 tbsp honey
FAT FRIENDLY	1 tbsp crushed walnuts
FREE FOODS	Water, tea

DINNER

Rosemary-Rubbed Salmon with Brown Rice and Steamed Artichoke

Steam artichoke over low heat for 30–40 min. Meanwhile, wash salmon with warm water and pat dry. Spray olive oil onto salmon fillet. Rub with finely chopped garlic, rosemary, salt and pepper. Squeeze a hint of lemon juice onto fish. Grill until fish flakes easily with a fork (about 4 min each side). Serve with brown rice and steamed artichoke.

Nutrition facts: 394 calories, 27 g protein, 56 g carbohydrates, 9 g fat

PROTEIN POWERED	90–115 g (3–4 oz) salmon (raw weight)
CARBOHYDRATE CONCENTRATED	100 g (3½ oz) cooked brown rice 1 medium steamed artichoke
FAT FRIENDLY	Extra virgin olive oil spray There are heart-healthy omega-3s in the salmon fillet.
FREE FOODS	1 tsp finely chopped garlic 1 tsp chopped rosemary Salt and ground black pepper Lemon wedges Water, tea

CHRISTINE'S NUTRITION NUGGETS Artichokes contain a compound known to help cleanse the liver of toxins . . . so eat up!

DAY 14
BREAKFAST

High-Protein Cereal with Berries
Make yourself a bowl and enjoy!

Nutrition facts: 353 calories, 30 g protein, 60 g carbohydrates, 3 g fat

PROTEIN POWERED	45 g (1½ oz) Kashi high-protein crunchy cereal 180 ml (6 fl oz) skimmed milk or soya milk
CARBOHYDRATE CONCENTRATED	Cereal should contain both carbs and protein. 60 g (2 oz) fresh blueberries
FAT FRIENDLY	It's in the cereal!
FREE FOODS	Water, tea, coffee

LUNCH

Sushi (Dining Out)
Order at your favourite sushi hot spot!

Nutrition facts: 326 calories, 22 g protein, 44 g carbohydrates, 4 g fat

PROTEIN POWERED	2 pieces salmon roll 2 pieces tuna roll* 2 pieces yellowtail roll *If pregnant, swap tuna for salmon. See Christine's Nutrition Nugget on page 133.
CARBOHYDRATE CONCENTRATED	Sushi is wrapped in rice, thus no need to add other carbs to this meal.
FAT FRIENDLY	⅕ diced avocado is usually found in sushi, so no need to add more fat to this meal.
FREE FOODS	Low-sodium soy sauce Wasabi 230 g (8 oz) steamed veggies Water, tea

CHRISTINE'S NUTRITION NUGGETS Wasabi is a spice known for its ulcer-fighting potential. A 2004 South Korean study suggests that Japanese horseradish can kill ulcer-causing *Helicobacter pylori* bacteria.

MID-AFTERNOON

Turkey and Cheese Roll-Up

Wrap deli slices around cheese sticks and dip into Dijon mustard. Enjoy with grapefruit and sweet cherries.

Nutrition facts: 359 calories, 24 g protein, 58 g carbohydrates, 10 g fat

PROTEIN POWERED	2 sticks light cheese strings 2 slices deli turkey
CARBOHYDRATE CONCENTRATED	1 large grapefruit 90 g (3 oz) fresh cherries
FAT FRIENDLY	No need to add fat because there is fat in the string cheese.
FREE FOODS	Dijon mustard Water, tea

DINNER

Sicilian-Style Chicken and Rice

See recipe on page 260.

Nutrition facts per serving: 414 calories, 33 g protein, 56 g carbohydrates, 6 g fat

PROTEIN POWERED	115 g (4 oz) skinless chicken breast
CARBOHYDRATE CONCENTRATED	Rice Tomato sauce
FAT FRIENDLY	Extra virgin olive oil
FREE FOODS	Garlic Green pepper Mushrooms Oregano Cayenne pepper Water, tea

CHAPTER 12

Supplemental Insurance

I have always recommended that my clients take three supplements daily: a multivitamin, a B-complex supplement and an omega-3 fatty acid supplement. As a nutritionist, I know this will prevent them from developing vitamin or mineral deficiencies, and I know the omega-3s will help combat bad fats. Clients will invariably ask me which brands I recommend, and my answer has always been the same: 'Any brand.'

Ironically, I haven't always followed my own recommendations. I used to feel that in order to set a good example, I should get all of my own nutrients from whole natural foods. If I ate a balanced diet from a large variety of sources, I thought, I would get 100 per cent of the nutrients my body needed, right?

Wrong.

I love to cook and I use all kinds of different fresh, whole, natural ingredients. I eat many different types of proteins and, overall, I assumed that my healthy variety would provide me with all the micronutrients my body needed. But in 2005, I had my hair coloured and I got a little wake-up call.

Before I knew it, my hair was brittle and broken. I would like to blame it on the colourist, but really my hair was too weak for the treatment. It was a frightening thing to see. I soon realized that my hair was not strong enough to withstand the straighteners every day, so I cut back to a few times a week. Still, my hair was coming out in clumps in the shower. It was so bad that I considered cutting it short or getting extensions or (God forbid) a wig. How did I get myself into this situation? I really thought I had been eating a great variety of foods, which should have been providing all the nutrients my hair needed. How could I be a 'healthy' nutritionist with my hair breaking off? Who wants to listen to a balding woman? When your hair isn't healthy, it makes you want to crawl into a dark cocoon and hide from the world.

I learned one of those painful lessons: vitamins and minerals are really no big deal – unless you aren't getting enough of them. I knew it was time to look into vitamin supplements.

Recommended daily amounts for essential nutrients were first introduced into the UK in the 1950s and represented guidelines for the amounts which would meet the needs of virtually everyone. They were intended to prevent deficiencies, optimize body stores and reduce the risk of disease.

In the early 1990s these were reviewed and reset by the Department of Health and by the European Community. They remain useful since although these days vitamin and mineral deficiencies are a lot less common, they still occur in certain groups of the population where needs are high or diet is poor. Vitamin and mineral content of supplements are usually expressed as a percentage of the EC RDA (Recommended Daily Allowance).

The symptoms of vitamin and mineral deficiencies are often subtle and hard to pinpoint, and sometimes they aren't much different from the minor complaints we experience every day, such as fatigue, confusion or emotional disturbances. Others are harder to ignore. Severe vitamin A deficiency can cause blindness (unlikely but possible), while a severe lack of niacin (vitamin B_3) can cause dementia. Those symptoms are extreme, but trust me, if you don't have the essential micronutrients you need, eventually your body will become sick.

The labels of many foods and supplements in the UK show the content of vitamins and minerals based on the EC RDA values – the levels needed to prevent disease. Clearly my hair was telling me that even if I was taking in these levels, it wasn't enough for vibrant health. The EC RDA also include upper limits on some of the vitamins to keep people from overdosing. You want to get enough but not too much. Here is the list of essential micronutrients. These are the vitamins and minerals for which the Department of Health has established the levels needed to assure good health.

VITAMINS	MINERALS
Vitamin A	Calcium
Thiamin (Vitamin B_1)	Chloride
Riboflavin (Vitamin B_2)	Chromium
Niacin (Vitamin B_3)	Copper
Pantothenic acid (Vitamin B_5)	Flouride
Vitamin B_6	Iodine
Folate (Vitamin B_9)	Iron
Vitamin B_{12}	Magnesium
Biotin	Manganese
Vitamin C	Molybdenum
Vitamin D	Phosphorus
Vitamin E	Potassium
Vitamin K	Selenium
	Sodium
	Zinc

At first I just wanted to know the vitamins that would help my hair. After dissecting the functions of each vitamin and mineral, I reached this conclusion: I needed *all* of them. When you start looking at the problems that can result from deficiencies and the benefits that come with proper nutrition, you see that every vitamin and mineral is important. I soon realized that it would be silly to take a specific set of vitamins for my hair and omit several others, possibly leading something else to go wrong. So I realized that the safest and smartest course of action was to meet all the RDAs, not just those that would specifically help my hair. You should do the same. Here are my recommendations.

Multivitamin: I recommend that all my clients take a general multivitamin. Choose a general multivitamin/mineral supplement which provides at least 15 nutrients but at levels at or below 150 per cent of the EC RDA. High doses of single nutrients are not necessary nor desirable and may put you at risk of adverse effects from excessive intakes. Some mineral compounds interfere with the absorption of others. For instance, high doses of calcium hinder iron absorption and high doses of zinc impair copper absorption. One multivitamin might claim to have it all, from A to Zinc, but your body might not be able to use all these nutrients at once. Others include only tiny amounts of one or more nutrient, and still other multivitamin formulas exclude iron. I suggest you choose a multivitamin/mineral that contains no iron unless you have been told specifically by a doctor to take iron. My eating plan will provide plenty without overdoing it.

Use caution when considering a multivitamin that advertises an 'add-on' ingredient that makes it different. This 'add-on' might include extracts from various herbs or enzymes. These other extracts are then marketed (carefully, so as not to violate the law) to deliver special benefits that are unique from those of the other multivitamins. Some of these claims are absolutely legitimate; most may not be. Those described as 'time released' or 'natural' vitamins are not absorbed any better than the comparable synthetic versions. Supplements with added enzymes have no benefit as they are destroyed by stomach acid and have no effect. High dose antioxidant supplements are not recommended, but a diet high in antioxidants is useful. If you take a supplement, don't forget to eat plenty of fresh fruit and vegetables (and wash them really well to get rid of any harmful residues).

B vitamins: B vitamins often act in concert with one another rather than individually. Researchers have a hard time pinpointing the effects of one or another B vitamin because often the nutrients are interdependent. This is one of the reasons I recommend that my clients take a B-complex supplement (a supplement that contains all of the B vitamins in one)

Skinny Chick 10-Week Transformation

HUSBAND AND WIFE TESTIMONIAL

NAME: MICHELLE E.
AGE: 37
TOTAL POUNDS LOST: 27 (12.2 kg)
TOTAL INCHES LOST: 37 (94 cm)

Most women I know who went off to university put on a stone (6.4 kilograms) in their first year; I put on nearly 2 stone (13 kilograms). That was when I first started gaining weight. I took it off, but I put it back on again, and it's a different story when you're in your thirties as far as losing weight goes.

I've tried every single weight loss programme on the market. After I got married, my husband and I both put on loads of weight, and I couldn't shed that weight no matter what I tried. Everything just made me put on more weight. I would lose 5 or 7 pounds (2.3–3.2 kilograms) and then I would crash and start eating and eating. I was like a drug addict, completely out of control. I would get moody, exhausted and collapse in the afternoon. All these failures sent me on bingeing sprees for days on end. I was very upset about it.

When I first started Christine's programme, she explained blood sugar and made a diagram about how what you eat affects your blood sugar. She explained that you need a balance, including carbs. The great thing was she gave me all these carbs I *wanted* to eat. I couldn't believe the size of my breakfast and my lunch. My husband would ask, 'Are you sure you can eat all that?' and I'd tell him, 'That's what Christine says!' So there I was, eating all the carbs people had told me not to eat, and feeling satisfied all day long. And I never once in 10 weeks was tempted to eat ice cream, or doughnuts or pastries

– which is a miracle for me. I never once binged, nor did I have the urge to binge. Now I feel wonderful. I feel vibrant. My body is thanking me. My husband's happy.

It's not even about vanity; it's about your health. At 37, I was already having weight-related health issues. I lived in tracksuit bottoms because that's all I could fit into. I didn't want to go to social functions. We live in Hollywood – my husband's a musician. Can you imagine being overweight and having to go into that world? It's a nightmare.

Before I started the programme, I began having medical problems. I had never before felt the health consequences of being overweight, and to be feeling that way at 37 was scary. If I hadn't found this programme, I can't imagine where I would be today or a year from today. I probably would be heading for an early grave.

Additional comments from Michelle's husband, Steve:

Just by eating what Michelle eats, I've lost over 2 stone (13 kilograms) without even trying. You stay full throughout the day. With a lot of diets, you find yourself starving and craving and crashing, and your blood sugar levels are all over the place. This is more of a lifestyle plan. You develop healthy habits almost in spite of yourself.

I wasn't planning to go on a diet. Michelle came home with this information one day, and I just jumped on board. Now our friends call us the incredible shrinking couple. And we're going to be eating this way for the rest of our lives.

rather than a product that contains one of the B vitamins alone. In other words, don't spend your money on a bottle of niacin capsules, biotin tablets or any other individual compound. Simply buy a B complex to include all of them at once for the best effect. B vitamins pass through the body quickly, so they need to be replenished daily. Choose a formula with no more than 150 per cent of the EC RDA of each of the B vitamin compounds.

Omega-3 fatty acids: My other primary recommendation is an omega-3 fatty acid supplement. Omega-3s are the good fats described in Chapter 9. They can help you lose weight, improve your mood, and lower your risk of heart disease. (I also believe they help make my skin and hair look shinier and healthier, but I suppose shiny hair is less important than a heart attack!) I recommend that everybody take a 1-gram-per-day omega-3 supplement. Make sure you buy yours from a reputable manufacturer that will provide certification of product purity if requested.

Additional supplementation: For some people there are occasions when insurance doses of certain nutrients might be of particular benefit. These include:

- a folic acid supplement of 400mcg daily taken before and until week 12 of pregnancy to prevent neural tube defects (spina bifida-type disorders)

- calcium supplements (together with at least 10mcg of Vitamin D daily) for people at risk of osteoporosis

- Vitamin D for breastfeeding mothers and infants under 2 years old

- Vitamin B12 for strict vegans

Other areas of supplementation may be beneficial, for example niacin and B group vitamins in heart disease; and B6 and/or magnesium in pre-menstrual tension. Research is under way in these areas.

You can find all of these supplements in any large supermarket or pharmacy. Alternatively, I have developed my own line of healthy supplements, with everything you need to help you achieve optimum health. They are available at www.christineavanti.com.

What about Weight Loss Supplements?

There are several weight loss pills available on the UK market and online which make unregulated and unsubstantiated claims. These are sold as food supplements rather than medicines and as such are currently not subject to the same strict controls and scrutiny.

Ephedra: Probably the biggest weight loss supplement to hit the market in recent memory was ephedra. Although it has been used for thousands of years, ephedra became extremely popular by the late 1990s as a dietary supplement. Tragically, it was found in the bodies of many people who died, including American footballer with the Minnesota Vikings Korey Stringer and Baltimore Orioles baseball pitcher Steve Bechler. Although ephedra was not specifically blamed for these deaths, both of these deaths were related to heatstroke, and ephedra is known to cause the body to overheat. The sale of ephedra has been intermittently banned in both the United States and the UK.

Green tea extract: Most of the manufacturers who made money selling ephedra products have switched to other formulas that are based on the next best weight loss ingredient: green tea extract, known as EGCg (Epigallocatechin gallate). In a study published in the *American Journal of Clinical Nutrition,* EGCg was found to increase energy expenditure and fat oxidation in humans. This study was quite impressive because it was able to prove that EGCg – rather than the caffeine in the tea – was responsible for the increase in metabolic rate. I love drinking green tea because of its antioxidant, anti-microbial and cholesterol-lowering activity. There are so many benefits from consuming tea that I could fill three more whole books on this single subject alone. However, I will only leave with a simple teaser: I recommend that you drink plenty of green tea. Should you take green tea extract supplements? I think they can be great; just don't expect miraculous results. It's fine to take a green tea-based supplement; just make sure it is from a good manufacturer and doesn't contain other ingredients that are harmful.

'Thermogenic' fat burners: From what I know, products that claim to be 'thermogenic' are largely based on the effects of caffeine derived from herbs such as yerba maté and guaraná. These fat burners increase your core body temperature and decrease appetite. Before becoming a certified nutritionist, I tried my fair share of fat burners with very high hopes. Most of them caused my heart to race and put me in a very bad mood. Another side effect I noticed was an increase in sugar cravings, because I was skipping meals. I recommend you avoid any supplement that claims to be a 'fat burner'. The most effective way to lose weight and burn fat is to follow the Skinny Chicks plan.

Carb blockers and fat blockers: I feel strongly that you should steer clear of any strategy that promises you can eat all you want and then alter the function of the body. You want your body to work as it is designed rather than 'blocking' the intended functions using foreign substances.

Thyroid increasers and cortisol suppressants: These products lack scientific evidence to back them up. Don't use yourself as a guinea pig. Instead, increase your metabolism naturally and suppress cortisol by eating according to the Skinny Chicks plan.

Hoodia: Hoodia seems to be everywhere you look these days. It is purported to suppress the appetite; however, I want you to have a large appetite because that means your metabolism is working. I don't recommend any supplements that interfere with your body's natural systems. Therefore, I don't recommend hoodia. Hoodia is one of the ingredients flooding the supplement market from what I call the junker companies. Don't be fooled by the dramatic claims made in ads from the junkers – there is no good evidence to support them.

Topical creams, gels and sprays: Fat must be released from within, and what is on your skin has no bearing whatsoever on the situation. More hooey.

The bottom line is that there are no great weight loss shortcuts on the market. Drinking green tea or taking a green tea extract supplement may help a little bit, and B-complex vitamins work together to help your metabolism. But most weight loss supplements are phony and don't help you lose anything except your hard-earned cash. My best advice is to take only supplements that have credible published scientific proof of benefits. You know the old saying, 'If it seems too good to be true . . . ' For the most current information, please visit my Web site at www.christineavanti.com, and follow the Skinny Chicks programme to get the healthiest body ever.

CHAPTER 13

Darnit, Get Your Lazy Butt on the Treadmill

As you have learned by now, I am an avid exerciser and have an extensive background in and understanding of the subject of fitness. In 1990, I became a certified aerobics instructor, and I taught aerobics as a hobby for 14 years until the demands of my nutrition consulting grew too pressing. In the mid-1990s, I was certified through California State University at Hayward for personal fitness coaching, and I also have qualifications in yoga, Spinning and cardiovascular conditioning.

I developed the Skinny Chicks programme so that even if you follow my eating plan and do no exercise whatsoever, your body will shed pounds of fat. Especially for people who are significantly overweight, it is hard to beat the effect of eating properly. For those who are 1½ stone (9.6 kilograms) overweight or less, it is a little harder to shed the fat. Regardless, I recommend that everybody incorporate some kind of workout into their daily routines because besides helping you lose weight, exercise has so many other health benefits that it should be an integral part of your Skinny Chicks lifestyle.

In this chapter, you will find three different workouts for three different levels of fitness: Beginner, Intermediate and Advanced. All three focus on the most effective movements for getting your body to ramp up its metabolism and burn body fat no matter what shape you are in.

Burning Body Fat

One of the biggest questions of the modern workout industry is which workouts cause the body to burn the most fat. There is a fat-melting workout promise on the cover of every fitness magazine every single month, yet you probably still don't know what type of exercise is really the best fat burner, do you? We all know that working out harder burns more calories, but are they calories from food, muscle or body fat? Well, you no longer have to wonder, because I am going to tell you the answer.

Cardiovascular exercise works the heart muscle and is the only type of exercise responsible for extreme fat burning. Here's why.

There are two types of muscle fibres in our bodies:

1. **Slow twitch:** These reddish muscle fibres mainly contract during steady, prolonged exercise, such as a chatty walk with your best friend. Slow-twitch fibre cells are loaded with microscopic organelles called mitochondria, within which a cellular metabolic process called the Krebs Cycle takes place. The Krebs Cycle, also known as the TCA Cycle or the Citric Acid Cycle, is responsible for kick-starting the fat-burning process. Therefore, you will burn mostly fat when using slow-twitch muscle fibres.

Through research, we know that slow-twitch muscle fibres are doing most of the work when you are exercising within your target heart rate zone, anywhere between 65 and 85 per cent of your maximal heart rate. (See below to calculate your target heart rate zone.)

2. **Fast twitch:** Fast-twitch muscle fibres mainly contract when intense, fast bursts of energy are needed – for example, when you need to get away from Godzilla and there is a huge rock wall in front of you! Fast-twitch muscle fibres are white because they do not contain as many of those precious little fat-burning mitochondrial organelles. Glycogen stores within muscle tissue mainly fuel fast-twitch muscle fibres. When the body uses glycogen stores for energy, muscle tissue is broken down and fat is hardly used, if it is used at all. Cyclist Lance Armstrong is an

excellent example of someone who focuses on training fast-twitch muscle fibres. Lance's goal is to increase speed and strength. We can all agree that Lance Armstrong does not need to burn fat, thus he can afford to train his fast-twitch muscle fibres all he wants.

Most of us have been convinced that we must be moving fast and furiously if we want to burn fat and lose weight. But many studies, such as the one reported in the *Scandinavian Journal of Medicine and Science in Sports* in 2006, have proven that slow-twitch muscle fibres burn more fat than fast-twitch fibres. Not only that, but all of the ladies from the Skinny Chicks test group exercised in this manner, and it yielded phenomenal results. That means you don't need to be sweating profusely and gasping for breath when you exercise – you just need to exert enough energy to stay within your target heart rate zone.

Enter Your Target Heart Rate Zone

It's easy to figure out your target heart rate (THR) zone. On most treadmills and exercise bikes in a gym, there is a simple chart showing how to work within your THR zone. Ask a member of staff to show you how to use it and you are on your way. You will be amazed to discover that it really isn't a hard pace to maintain. Read a magazine, watch some trashy TV, improve your mind by reading a good book and burn away fat at an easy-to-maintain pace. *This* is the pace that makes the body draw upon fat storage for energy.

If you are not using the exercise bike or the treadmill and you want to work in your THR, there are two options. One is to buy a heart rate monitor. These are inexpensive and available at any sports shop. They can be programmed to beep when you are working too fast or too slow. They are a really cool and effective product, and I highly recommend them. The other option is to use the following equation:

Subtract your age from 220. For instance, if you are 40 years old:

```
220   Take the number  220
- 40  subtract your age
─────────────────────────────
= 180  your Max Heart Rate (MHR)
```

Then take your MHR and multiply it by 65 per cent and 85 per cent to get the lower and upper limits of your THR zone.

Lower limit: multiply your MHR by 65%   180 x 65% = 117
Upper limit: multiply your MHR by 85%   180 x 85% = 153

So if you are 40 years old, your fat-burning target heart rate zone is between 117 heartbeats per minute and 153 heartbeats per minute. What I tell people to do is to look at that lower number; in this case, let's round it up to 120. This means that if your heart beats 12 times in 6 seconds, you are in your zone (there are 60 seconds in a minute, so if your heart beats 12 times in 6 seconds, it is beating 120 times in 60 seconds).

Now, how do you measure this without any equipment? Simple: you stop walking (or cycling, dancing or whatever) and you find your pulse by placing two fingers flat on the side of your neck. When you feel your pulse, count the beats while watching a clock for 6 seconds. Then multiply the number of beats by 10. So if you counted 13 beats, you multiply by 10 to get 130. Bingo! You are well within your THR (117 to 153 in the example above).

I'll do the breakdown for you so that you can make sure you get into your minimum THR:

Age 20 to 33:   Aim for at least 13 heartbeats in 6 seconds
(130 beats per minute, or BPM)

Age 34 to 46:   Aim for at least 12 heartbeats in 6 seconds
(120 BPM)

Age 47 to 56:   Aim for at least 11 heartbeats in 6 seconds
(110 BPM)

Age 57 to 70:   Aim for at least 10 heartbeats in 6 seconds
(100 BPM)

Age 71 and up: Aim for at least 9 heartbeats in 6 seconds
(90 BPM)

For more examples, pictures and a THR calculator, please visit my Web site at www.christineavanti.com.

Skinny Chick Chat

· ·

DEAR CHRISTINE: I've heard some personal trainers say that you should work out first thing in the morning before breakfast. What's your opinion?

MONA B.

MONA: Many personal trainers say to work out early in the morning on an empty stomach and then to avoid eating for an hour afterwards to burn as much fat as possible. I can see why this workout concept is attractive to busy individuals. The problem is that the body, having depleted Tank 1 (blood sugar) and Tank 2 (glycogen stores), is accessing muscle tissue for fuel along with body fat. There is no question that you will work off some fat. But most people who put their bodies in this kind of nutrient deficit will be working out while they have low blood sugar levels, which will cause them to overeat later in the day and reverse their gains (or in this case, losses). It would be better to have a small, balanced meal (such as low-fat Greek yogurt and a little low-fat granola) before the workout to keep the metabolism stable.

You need a workout that won't interrupt your eating plan. You need to eat a reasonable amount of a balance of nutrients at 4-hour intervals (remember your ABCs). So this means you should not work out on an empty stomach; rather, you should work out at any time during the day that doesn't interrupt your eating schedule. If you want to get your workout done early in the morning, simply grab a quick breakfast before you go.

EAT WELL, CHRISTINE

I'm not the only nutrition and fitness expert who strongly believes that exercise within your target heart rate zone is most effective for fat burning. Mark Twight, the owner of a training facility called Gym Jones in Salt Lake City in the US, used this principle to get the cast of the movie *300* into ultra-fit shape in 3 months through hard work and diet without any performance-enhancing drugs.

Although this concept may seem to defy logic, here's why it works: as we know, 1 gram of fat contains 9 units of energy (calories), whereas 1 gram of sugar (glucose) – which is found in muscle tissue – has only 4 units of energy. Because fat is a denser source of energy, you don't need to work as hard when you are using fat for fuel.

Don't 'Dis' Your Muscles

Just because you're looking to burn fat doesn't mean you can ignore your muscles altogether. You need muscle to burn fat. Remember that a 10-stone (64-kilogram) woman with nice muscle tone is much smaller than the same woman with little muscle but a lot of fat, because the fat takes up much more space than the same weight in muscle. The best way to build muscle is through resistance training, exercises that use an opposing force to strengthen muscles. Resistance can be supplied by free weights (e.g. dumbbells), elastic bands or even your own body weight.

You don't have to become a body builder or end up with an unnaturally muscular physique. But to look your best, you should aim for a toned, lean body. Not only does that improve your appearance, it helps you lose weight as well, because muscle burns fat 24/7 – even when you're resting. Your resting metabolic rate increases when your muscle mass increases. The more muscle you have, the faster your metabolism works. So you need to do some resistance training to build muscle to burn fat around the clock. Increased bone mass and density is another great perk associated with strength training.

Assuming that you are eating correctly and working out between meals, what is the best workout for burning body fat? The perfect fat-burning workout would be a combination of weight training and cardiovascular exercises, such as those listed on the following page.

Recommended Weekly Workout Schedule

My workout recommendations are broken down into three categories: Beginner, Intermediate and Advanced. At each level, my workouts will focus your efforts on fat burning.

Beginner Workout — *For Non-active People*

This beginners' exercise plan is for people who have scarcely ever been inside a gym or who haven't worked out in more than 6 months. It allows the body to warm up slowly and get accustomed to using muscles that haven't been active for a while. It is easy and quick, yet it is very effective in getting the whole body involved and active. Remember that most of the people in the gym are not getting the benefit of a great nutrition plan like you are, so you will soon have amazing results.

If you are a total beginner, I highly recommend that you work with a personal trainer or other fitness professional the first time you do any of these exercises. Always consult your doctor if you have any doubts about your condition for exercising. When you exercise, it is important to work within the appropriate level of intensity for your health. For a beginner, the intensity level is not nearly as important as maintaining proper form. I recommend you work out at approximately 40 to 50 per cent intensity. Aim to exercise within your target heart rate zone when doing cardio. If you have never worked out regularly, it is very important that you exercise for no more than 10 minutes on your first day. Here is a safe and effective exercise schedule for a beginner:

Skinny Chicks Cardiovascular Progression Chart

WEEK	DAY 1	DAY 2	DAY 3	DAY 4	DAY 5	DAY 6	DAY 7
1	10 min	15 min	20 min	25 min	30 min	Off	Off
2	30 min	30 min	30 min	30 min	30 min	Off	Off
3	30 min	35 min	35 min	35 min	35 min	Off	Off
4	35 min	35 min	35 min	35 min	35 min	Off	Off
5	35 min	35 min	Continue doing cardio a minimum of 4 days per week at 35 min per session to build up your cardiovascular endurance safely.				

The type of exercise you choose might include any of the following:

- Walking on a treadmill
- Walking outside
- Riding an exercise bike
- Swimming
- Elliptical trainer
- Stairclimber
- Rowing machine
- Low-impact aerobics (within your target heart rate zone only!)
- Spinning (within your target heart rate zone only!)
- Any other form of exercise that you enjoy and that involves the large muscles of the hips, thighs and buttocks, such as salsa dancing, hiking, mountain biking, etc. I call this 'fun' cardio.

Each cardiovascular exercise session should be performed in your target heart rate zone. In order to maximize the efficiency of your cardiovascular exercise, I highly recommend that you wear a heart rate monitor to ensure that you are exercising within your target heart rate zone at all times.

BEGINNER MUSCLE TONING AT HOME

Once you are comfortable with performing cardiovascular exercise at least four times per week for a minimum of 1 month, you can begin to incorporate some light toning exercises, such as the ones below. Having been a gym junkie for the past 18 years, I've learned which exercises benefit specific areas of the female anatomy most. So, for the Skinny Chicks workout, I have listed my favourites:

Reverse Lunge

Benefit: It lifts a sagging butt faster then any other exercise I've ever known (and I've tried them all).

Step 1: Stand in a doorway and place your hand on the door frame for balance.

Step 2: Start with both of your feet together. Step backwards with one foot as far as you can. Bend both knees until the back knee almost touches the floor. It is important that your front knee be directly above your ankle joint. If your forward knee pushes past your ankle joint, you will put too much pressure on the front knee and can cause injury. Just tell yourself, your knees cannot be over your toes.

Step 3: Go back to the starting position by pressing through your front foot; focus on pushing through your heel. You should notice your glutes (butt) contracting . . . this is what you want.

Step 4: Alternate with the other leg.

Repetitions: Do a total of 20 alternating reverse lunges 3 days a week, and watch your behind get firm and lifted in no time!

Standing Calf Raise
Benefit: Nice calves that will look fantastic with a skirt and pair of high heels!

Step 1: Stand in a doorway with your feet hip-width apart, and place one hand on the door frame for balance.

Step 2: Slowly lift your heels off the floor as high as you can. Hold that position for 5 seconds, then lower back to the floor.

Repetitions: Do 3 sets of 10 reps. Don't forget to stretch out your calves afterwards, by placing your toes against the wall while keeping your heel on the floor. Stretch one foot at a time, and lean forwards. I often do these in the bathroom as I'm getting ready for work.

Wall or Worktop Press-up
Benefit: Lifts a sagging chest, so everything will start to look perky again.

Step 1: Standing up straight, place both hands on a wall or worktop. Your hands should be slightly more than shoulder-width apart. Your feet should be about 30 to 60 centimetres (1 to 2 feet) away from the wall, so that you are leaning towards the wall at an angle. Bend your elbows and lean into the wall or worktop.

Step 2: Contract your mid-section (core) and press yourself away from the wall or countertop until your arms are straight. Don't slouch in your lower back; stay as straight as you can.

Repetitions: Do a total of 3 sets of 10 press-ups, 3 days a week.

Triceps Dip

Benefit: Gets rid of those flabby bat wings on the backs of your arms.

Step 1: Sit on the edge of your bath or a sturdy kitchen chair that won't tip over, and place your hands on either side of you, just under your buttocks.

Step 2: Straighten your arms and shift your body away from the edge so you can dip your buttocks down towards the floor. Place your feet as far away from your seat as you can, dig your heels into the floor and point your toes to the ceiling.

Step 3: Dip your rear down by bending through your elbows, then press yourself back up. You should feel the backs of your arms contracting. The muscles contracting are your triceps (the 'wing' part is called fat).

Repetitions: Do 3 sets of 10 dips, 3 times a week.

Ball or Floor Crunch

Benefit: Get back that six-pack that became a one-pack at some point between the ages of 19 and 39!

If you have a large exercise ball, you can perform 'ball crunches'; if not, floor crunches work really well, too.

Ball Crunch: Using a medium-sized body ball, sit on top of the ball with your feet placed firmly on the floor. Next, walk your feet forwards, and as you move forwards, allow your rear to move forwards too, so that your lower back is resting on the ball. Cross your arms over your chest, engage your lower stomach area and crunch forwards. Make sure you can feel your abs during each crunch.

Floor Crunch: Lie full length on a mat or floor with a padded surface. Slide your feet halfway up towards your body, and place your hands

behind your upper neck. Crunch forwards, keeping your chin up. Do
not let your chin cave in to your neck; this ensures that you will be
contracting your abs to lift you up. Come up one-quarter of the way,
then release back to the floor. Repeat.

Repetitions: Start out slowly at 3 sets of 10 reps. You should be able
to increase to 3 sets of 20 ab crunches fairly quickly.

BEGINNER CARDIO/TONING WORKOUT AT A GLANCE

Week 1 – Beginner

DAY 1	DAY 2	DAY 3	DAY 4	DAY 5	DAY 6	DAY 7
Cardio and muscle toning	Cardio	Cardio and muscle toning	Off	Off	Cardio and muscle toning	Cardio

At Home Light Upper-Body Workout – Beginner

SET	MUSCLE GROUP	EXERCISE	REPS	INTENSITY	REST
1	Chest, shoulders, and back	Wall or Worktop Press-up (page 183)	10	50%	30 sec
2		Wall or Worktop Press-up	10	50%	30 sec
3		Wall or Worktop Press-up	10	50%	30 sec
4	Triceps	Triceps Dip (page 184)	10	50%	30 sec
5		Triceps Dip	10	50%	30 sec
6		Triceps Dip	10	50%	30 sec
	Total time:	About 7 min			

At Home Light Lower-Body Workout – Beginner

SET	MUSCLE GROUP	EXERCISE	REPS	INTENSITY	REST
1	Quads (fronts of your thighs), buttocks, hamstrings	Reverse Lunge (page 182)	20	50%	1 min
2		Standing Calf Raise (page 183)	10	50%	30 sec
3	Calves	Standing Calf Raise	10	50%	30 sec
4		Standing Calf Raise	10	50%	30 sec
5		Ball or Floor Crunch (page 184)	10	50%	30 sec
6	Abs	Crunch	15	50%	30 sec
7		Crunch	20	50%	30 sec
8		Crunch	20	50%	30 sec
	Total time:	About 30 min			

Week 2 – Repeat Week 1 Schedule, but increase intensity and duration of cardio workout according to the chart on page 181.

Week 3 – Repeat Week 2 Schedule, but increase intensity a little more and increase cardio time as indicated in the chart on page 181.

Intermediate Workout – *For People Who Are Comfortable in a Gym or Have Completed 3 Weeks of the Beginner Workout*

Now we are starting to get a little more serious. The equipment in the gym can be a great aid to getting in shape, but it is important that you learn how to use it properly to avoid injury. Safety first!

Before beginning the workout below, get into position and do each movement *without weights* for 15 reps. This is very important because it warms up your muscles and the joints. If you feel any strange pains while doing the movement without weights, stop immediately and seek advice from a knowledgeable personal trainer or fitness professional. *Do not* try the movement with weights if you feel pain without weights. If you did not feel any strange pains, go ahead and try the workout with very light weights (1- or 2.5-pound/500-gram or 1-kilogram dumbbells for most exercises, no weights for the leg press) for the first set. In this phase, you are simply trying to get your muscles moving and stretching. During your rest, always stretch the muscles you are working out.

If you miss a workout, don't skip ahead; simply pick up where you left off.

Week 1 – Intermediate

DAY 1	45 min cardio or fast walk around the local area
DAY 2	Weights: 30-Minute Upper-Body Workout (page 188) 30 min cardio
DAY 3	45 min cardio or fast walk around the local area
DAY 4	45 min cardio or fast walk around the local area
DAY 5	Off
DAY 6	Weights: 30-Minute Lower-Body Workout (page 189) 30 min cardio
DAY 7	Off

30-Minute Upper-Body Workout — Intermediate

SET	MUSCLE GROUP	EXERCISE	REPS	INTENSITY	REST
1		Dumbbell Bench Press (page 190)	15	50%	45 sec
2	Chest	Dumbbell Bench Press	15	50%	45 sec
3		Pushup (page 190)	10–15	50%	90 sec
4		Seated Overhead Shoulder Press (page 190)	15	50%	45 sec
5	Shoulders	Seated Overhead Shoulder Press	15	50%	45 sec
6		Side Lateral Raise (page 191)	15	50%	90 sec
7		Seated Machine Row (page 191)	15	50%	45 sec
8	Back	Seated Machine Row	15	50%	45 sec
9		Lat Machine Pulldown (page 191)	15	50%	45 sec
10		Lat Machine Pulldown	15	50%	90 sec
11		Triceps Cable Pushdown (page 192)	15	50%	45 sec
12	Triceps	Triceps Cable Pushdown	15	50%	45 sec
13		Seated Dumbbell Extension (page 192)	15	50%	45 sec
14		Seated Dumbbell Extension	15	50%	90 sec
15		Seated Dumbbell Curl (page 192)	15	50%	45 sec
16	Biceps	Seated Dumbbell Curl	15	50%	45 sec
17		Standing Barbell Curl (page 193)	15	50%	45 sec
18		Standing Barbell Curl	15	50%	45 sec
	Total time:	About 30 min			

30-Minute Lower-Body Workout – Intermediate

SET	MUSCLE GROUP	EXERCISE	REPS	INTENSITY	REST
1		Leg Press (page 194)	20	50%	1 min
2	Quads	Leg Press	20	50%	1 min
3		Leg Press	20	50%	2 min
4		Dumbbell Reverse Lunge (page 194)	16	50%	1 min
5	Buttocks	Dumbbell Reverse Lunge	16	50%	1 min
6		Dumbbell Reverse Lunge	16	50%	2 min
7		Lying Leg Curl (page 194)	20	50%	45 sec
8	Hamstrings	Lying Leg Curl	20	50%	45 sec
9		Lying Leg Curl	20	50%	45 sec
10	Calves	Calf Raise (page 195)	20	50%	45 sec
11		Calf Raise	20	50%	2 min
12		Ball or Floor Crunch (page 195)	20	50%	45 sec
13	Abs	Crunch	20	50%	45 sec
14		Crunch	20	50%	45 sec
15		Crunch	20	50%	45 sec
	Total time:	About 30 min			

Week 2 – Repeat Week 1 Schedule, but increase intensity in the gym to 60 per cent maximum effort.

Week 3 – Repeat Week 2 Schedule, but increase intensity in the gym to 70 per cent maximum effort and increase fun cardio or walking on Tuesday and Saturday to 45 minutes.

INTERMEDIATE AND ADVANCED EXERCISES

Dumbbell Bench Press
Benefits: Strengthens your chest, shoulders and triceps.

Step 1: Grab a dumbbell in each hand, lie flat on a bench with your feet flat on the floor, and tilt your pelvis forwards so that each of your vertebrae are touching the bench. (If you cannot feel each of your vertebrae touching the bench, it is OK to place your feet on the bench instead of the floor. However, the first position is the safest.)

Step 2: Contract your abdominal muscles inwards (this ensures a strong core). Next, press the dumbbells upwards with your elbows at your sides, until your arms are extended.

Step 3: Lower the weights to the sides of your upper chest until you feel a slight stretch in your chest or shoulders. Repeat.

Press-up
Benefits: Strengthens your chest, anterior deltoids, and triceps.

Step 1: Kneel on all fours with your wrists directly under shoulders, your arms straight and your knees under your hips. Move your hands slightly further apart than shoulder width and tuck your hips forwards so your torso forms a straight line from your head to your knees.

Step 2: Bend your elbows and lower your body towards the floor until your elbows are aligned with your shoulders.

Step 3: Push up to the starting position and repeat.

Seated Overhead Shoulder Press
Benefit: Strengthens your deltoids (shoulder muscles).

Step 1: Sit on a 90-degree-angle, back-supported bench and grab two dumbbells. Bring the dumbbells up to the fronts of your shoulders, with your palms forwards and your abs tight for a strong core.

Step 2: Press the dumbbells up and overhead in an arch motion and softly tap the dumbbells at the top.

Step 3: Lower the dumbbells slowly and repeat.

Side Lateral Raise

Benefit: Strengthens your medial deltoids (the middle muscle of your shoulders).

Step 1: Stand with your knees slightly bent and tighten your abdominals. Hold the dumbbells at your sides with your palms facing your thighs.

Step 2: Slowly raise your arms out laterally from your sides. Focus on lifting through your elbows rather than your hands (this will cause you to contract your medial deltoids more), and pause when the dumbbells are at shoulder height.

Step 3: Slowly lower the dumbbells and repeat.

Seated Machine Row

Benefits: Strengthens your back and biceps.

Step 1: Sit at a cable rowing machine with a small triangle handle attached to the cable. Place your feet firmly on the foot dock, grasp the handle with both hands, and slowly sit up with your back straight and your shoulders back in their sockets.

Step 2: Next, pull or row the handle in to your abs, moving your elbows as far back as possible.

Step 3: Slowly release to return the handle to the starting position, and repeat.

Lat Machine Pulldown

Benefits: Strengthens your latissimus dorsi (back muscles) and biceps.

Step 1: Sit at a pulldown machine with your legs snugly under the kneepads. With your feet firmly on the floor, grasp the wide bar with an overhand grip. Your hands should be twice your shoulder width apart (as wide as possible).

Step 2: Slightly arch your back as you pull the bar down to the top of your chest.

Step 3: Focus on keeping your elbows below the bar, pause and contract your back muscles, and slowly raise the bar back to the starting position. Do not lean back using your body weight to pull the bar down. If you notice that you are doing this, lighten the weight.

Triceps Cable Pushdown
Benefit: Strengthens your triceps.

Step 1: Stand facing a high cable pulley with your knees slightly bent, your shoulders back in their sockets, your chest forwards, your elbows in line with your shoulders close to your rib cage and your arms bent.

Step 2: Straighten your arms, pressing down towards your thighs.

Step 3: Keeping your elbows close to your rib cage, bend your arms upwards and repeat.

Seated Dumbbell Extension (a.k.a. French Press)
Benefit: Strengthens your triceps.

Step 1: Start with a dumbbell weight that you can hold above your head using two hands. Sit on a bench with your back straight, your feet firmly on the floor and your abs tight.

Step 2: Grasp the dumbbell underhand around the shaft with both hands for a firm grip and press it above your head, contracting the backs of your arms.

Step 3: Lower slowly and repeat.

Seated Dumbbell Curl
Benefit: Strengthens your biceps.

Step 1: Sit on a 90-degree-angle, back-supported bench and grab two dumbbells. With both feet firmly on the floor and your abs tight, hold the dumbbells using an underhand grip.

Step 2: Starting in the down position, keep your elbows close to your rib cage, bend at the elbows and curl the weights up to the fronts of your shoulders.

Step 3: Lower slowly and repeat.

Standing Barbell Curl

Benefit: Strengthens your biceps.

Step 1: Stand straight with your shoulders back and your knees slightly bent. Grab a barbell using an underhand grip.

Step 2: Starting with the barbell in front of your thighs in the down position, keep your elbows close to your rib cage, bend at the elbows and curl the weights up. The barbell should stay close to your body as it travels upwards to the fronts of your shoulders.

Step 3: Lower slowly and repeat.

Incline Dumbbell Fly

Benefit: Strengthens your inner pectoral muscles (they make a beautiful line down the middle of the chest).

Step 1: Lie on an incline bench angled at 60 degrees, with your feet firmly on the floor and your abs tight. Hold a dumbbell in each hand above your chest. Your arms should be straight, and your palms should mirror each other.

Step 2: Next, bend your elbows out and down to align the dumbbells with your shoulders.

Step 3: Lift up and repeat.

Incline Dumbbell Press

Benefit: Strengthens your pectoral muscles.

Step 1: Lie on an incline bench angled at 60 degrees, with your feet firmly on the floor and your abs tight. Hold a dumbbell in each hand above your chest, with your arms straight and your palms facing away from your body.

Step 2: Next, bend your elbows downwards until the dumbbells are aligned with your shoulders.

Step 3: Press up and lightly tap the dumbbells together upon extension. Repeat.

Leg Press

Benefits: Strengthens your quadriceps, hamstrings and gluteal muscles.

Step 1: Sit on a 45-degree-angled leg press machine (most gyms have these), and place your feet on the platform, hip-width apart.

Step 2: Press the platform up, release the dock safety lever, and grasp the side handles. Now lower the sled by bending your knees until they are slightly beyond a 90-degree angle.

Step 3: Press up to the starting position, and focus on pressing through your heels as opposed to the balls of your feet. This helps to even the work between your quads, hamstrings and glutes. Repeat.

Dumbbell Reverse Lunge

Benefits: Strengthens your gluteal muscles, quads and hamstrings.

Step 1: Stand with your feet hip-width apart and grab a dumbbell in each hand. Let the dumbbells hang down at your sides, near your outer thighs.

Step 2: Begin by stepping one foot back behind you. Reach your foot back as far as you can. You should feel a stretch in the hip flexor muscle of your back leg.

Step 3: Lower yourself slowly, stopping just before your back knee touches the floor. Bring your back foot forwards and repeat with the other leg.

Lying Leg Curl (a.k.a. Hamstring Curl)

Benefits: Strengthens your hamstrings and glutes.

Step 1: On a hamstring machine (found at most gyms), lie on your stomach, hook your feet under the circular ankle pad and flex your feet (do not point your toes).

Step 2: Slowly curl your legs up and in towards your buttocks in an arching motion.

Step 3: Squeeze your hamstrings and glutes, then slowly release back to the starting position. Repeat.

Calf Raise

Benefit: Strengthens your calf muscles.

Step 1: Grab a dumbbell in each hand and let them hang at your sides. Stand with your feet hip-width apart and your knees slightly bent.

Step 2: Slowly lift your heels off the floor as high as you can.

Step 3: Hold the position for 5 seconds, then lower your heels back to the floor. Repeat.

Ball Crunch

Benefit: Strengthens your abs.

Step 1: Using a medium-size body ball, sit on top of the ball with your feet placed firmly on the floor.

Step 2: Next, walk your feet forwards, and as you move forwards, allow your rear to move forwards too, so that your lower back is resting on the ball.

Step 3: Cross your arms over your chest, engage your lower stomach area and crunch forwards. Make sure you can feel your abs during each crunch.

Floor Crunch

Benefit: Strengthens your abs.

Step 1: Lay full length on a mat or floor with a padded surface. Slide your feet halfway up towards your body and place your hands behind your upper neck.

Step 2: Crunch forwards, keeping your chin up. Do not let your chin cave in to your neck; this ensures that you will be contracting your abs to lift you up.

Step 3: Come up one-quarter of the way, then release back to the floor. Repeat.

Skinny Chicks
Workout Guidelines

• Do cardio in your target heart rate zone (not too fast).

• Find an activity that you love to do — your fun cardio.

• Do your fun cardio immediately after weight training to better access body fat for energy.

• Do weight training or other resistance training to increase muscle tone. You will burn calories (and fat) during the workout and throughout the day.

• If you are just beginning, get a personal trainer or fitness professional to demonstrate the exercises and machinery for you.

• Work your way gradually from very light weights to heavier weights to increase your intensity.

• Always stretch the muscles you are working between sets.

• After a few weeks, you should strive to reach 100 per cent maximum exertion in your weight lifting workouts, but keep your fun cardio within your THR zone.

Advanced Workout – *For Active People or Beginners Who Have Completed 4 Weeks of the Intermediate Plan*

The next stage is for people who are ready to step it up to a level that begins to reshape the body. By now you should have worked out some options for your cardio. You've also warmed up your muscles and joints so that weight training can be increased. You only have to work out 3 days per week, but I have stacked the workouts so that you are getting the maximum fat burning benefit. If you like, you may do the cardio on the off days to fit your schedule better, but it is best to do it as a continuous block to access the most fat storage for energy. Try to do the whole routine at least once at the weekend when you have more time.

Week 2 is identical to Week 1 except that the upper- and lower-body weight training circuits are alternated. If you look at the table beginning on page 198, you'll see that on the first set of each new muscle group, the intensity is always 50 per cent, meaning that you should be able to perform the exercise with a bit of strain . . . but not zero strain. This is just a 'warmup' set to get your muscles and joints prepared for the heavy workload to come in the next set, and it uses a light weight and more reps. As the weeks go on and you grow more comfortable with your weights, increase the intensity of your last set for each muscle group by grabbing a slightly heavier weight. As an alternative to doing the workout, you may do a body sculpting class.

Week 1 – Advanced

DAY 1	DAY 2	DAY 3	DAY 4	DAY 5	DAY 6	DAY 7
Weights: 45-Minute Lower-Body Workout (page 189) at 85% of maximum effort		Weights: 45-Minute Upper-Body Workout (page 188) at 85% max effort		Off	Weights: 45-Minute Lower-Body Workout at 85% max effort	
30–60 min of cardio	1 hr cardio	1 hr cardio	30–60 min of cardio		1 hr cardio immediately after gym	1 hr cardio

Week 2 – Advanced

	DAY 1	DAY 2	DAY 3	DAY 4	DAY 5	DAY 6	DAY 7
	Weights: 45-Minute Lower-Body and Abs Workout at 85% of max effort	Off	Weights: 45-Minute Upper-Body Workout at 85% of max effort	Off	Off	Weights: 45-Minute Lower-Body and Abs Workout at 85% of max effort	Off
	1 hr fun cardio – do immediately after gym or tomorrow		1 hr fun cardio – do immediately after gym or tomorrow			1–2 hrs fun cardio immediately after gym	

45-Minute Upper-Body Workout – Advanced

SET	MUSCLE GROUP	EXERCISE	REPS	INTENSITY	REST
1		Dumbbell Bench Press (page 190)	20	50%	45 sec
2		Dumbbell Bench Press	12	85%	45 sec
3	Chest	Dumbbell Bench Press	12	85%	45 sec
4		Incline Dumbbell Fly (page 193)	12	85%	45 sec
5		Incline Dumbbell Fly	10	85–100%	90 sec
6		Seated Overhead Shoulder Press (page 190)	20	50%	45 sec
7		Incline Dumbbell Press (page 193)	12	85%	45 sec
8	Shoulders	Incline Dumbbell Press	12	85%	45 sec
9		Side Lateral Raise (page 191)	12	85%	45 sec
10		Side Lateral Raise	10	85–100%	90 sec
11		Seated Machine Row (page 191)	20	50%	45 sec
12		Seated Machine Row	15	85%	45 sec
13	Back	Seated Machine Row	15	85%	45 sec
14		Lat Machine Pulldown (page 191)	15	85%	45 sec
15		Lat Machine Pulldown	12	85–100%	90 sec

SET	MUSCLE GROUP	EXERCISE	REPS	INTENSITY	REST
16		Triceps Cable Pushdown (page 192)	20	50%	45 sec
17		Triceps Cable Pushdown	15	85%	45 sec
18	Triceps	Seated Dumbbell Extension (page 192)	15	85%	45 sec
19		Seated Dumbbell Extension	15	85%	45 sec
20		Seated Dumbbell Extension	12	85–100%	90 sec
21		Seated Dumbbell Curl (page 192)	15	50%	45 sec
22		Seated Dumbbell Curl	15	85%	45 sec
23	Biceps	Standing Barbell Curl (page 193)	15	85%	45 sec
24		Standing Barbell Curl	15	85%	45 sec
25		Standing Barbell Curl	12	85–100%	
	Total time:	About 30–40 min			

45-Minute Lower-Body and Abs Workout – Advanced

SET	MUSCLE GROUP	EXERCISE	REPS	INTENSITY	REST
1		Leg Press (page 194)	30	50%	1 min
2	Quads	Leg Press	20	85%	1 min
3		Leg Press	15	85–100%	2 min
4		Dumbbell Reverse Lunge (page 194)	20	50%	1 min
5	Buttocks	Dumbbell Reverse Lunge	16	85%	1 min
6		Dumbbell Reverse Lunge	16	85%	1 min
7		Lying Leg Curl (page 194)	25	50%	1 min
8	Hamstrings	Lying Leg Curl	16	85%	1 min
9		Lying Leg Curl	12	85–100%	2 min
10	Calves	Calf Raise (page 195)	20	85%	1 min
11		Calf Raise	20	85–100%	1 min

(continued)

SET	MUSCLE GROUP	EXERCISE	REPS	INTENSITY	REST
12		Ball Crunch (page 195)	20	85%	1 min
13		Ball Crunch	20	85%	1 min
14	Abs	Ball Crunch	20	85–100%	1 min
15		Floor Crunch (page 195)	20	85%	1 min
16		Floor Crunch	20	85%	1 min
17		Floor Crunch	20	85–100%	1 min
	Total time:	About 30–40 min			

Weeks 3 and 4 – Repeat Weeks 1 and 2 but gradually increase intensity level.

Don't forget to keep your body well fuelled for your workouts to get the most from your time in the gym. If you are eating according to the Skinny Chicks plan, your body should have all the nutrients it needs for energy. But on days when you are not feeling 100 per cent, I recommend taking a B vitamin-based energy boost before your workout.

Skinny Chick 10-Week Transformation

NAME: CASEY F.

AGE: 47

TOTAL POUNDS LOST: 17 (7.7 kg)

TOTAL INCHES LOST: 21 (53.3 cm)

I remember being body conscious when I was at school. I was very involved in sports and had a muscular build. I joined the cheerleading squad, but as soon as I put that little skirt on, I felt different from the others. I wished I had skinny little legs like they did.

My involvement in sports grew throughout my teenage years, and I began to embrace my muscular build. I always managed to make working out a priority. When I went to university, I became very interested in health food – I actually became kind of fanatical about it – and I was compulsive about everything I ate. I managed to stay very slim until my first child was born, when I was 35, but I found it very difficult to lose the weight once the baby was born.

From that point on, things began to change. Life got in the way, and it wasn't all about me any more. My workouts became sporadic at best; my eating habits changed. I was practically starving myself. I began to skip meals and eat foods that were higher in fats and calories. And then I found the Skinny Chicks programme. Since following Christine's guidelines, I have changed from head to toe. My face is thinner and looks much younger. I have a flatter stomach and my love handles are gone. My legs are thinner and don't rub together when I walk any more. But the greatest impact has been on my energy levels. I used to go to bed exhausted, sleep for 8 hours and wake up exhausted. Now I pop out of bed and feel great. I embrace each day and I am much more productive.

PART IV

SKINNY CHICKS

IN THE

REAL WORLD

CHAPTER 14

Skinny Chicks Have
Their Ups and Downs

Here is something you might want to know. Once you have settled into your eating plan and your blood sugar levels have stabilized (anywhere from 3 days to a few weeks into your plan), your body will begin to burn fat steadily. Nearly every one of my clients tells me they feel better than they have in years, with calm, steady energy and a healthy appetite. Once you eat on my plan for a while, you get very addicted to having a consistent, stable energy level, and it will be very apparent when you don't eat properly. A single massive sugar binge can upset your metabolism and blood sugar stability for several days. If, one night, you decide to throw it all to the wind and have a psycho pizza pig-out, you might feel lethargic for the next few days and have no desire to eat on your schedule. When there is something difficult going on in your life, like a break-up or a work deadline, you may find it hard to resist saying 'to hell with it' and just eat takeaways and ice cream all weekend.

What many people do after a binge is make up for it by trying to eat as little as possible the next day. They revert to old fad diets and doubt the validity of real nutritional science: the ABCs. Somewhere in the back of their minds, they still hold on to the belief that the *real* way to lose weight is either to starve themselves or to avoid all carbs. But all this does is slow your metabolism, deprive your body of required nutrients and set you up for another binge – just as holding your breath underwater sets you up to pop to the surface for air. You can't hold your breath for ever, and you can't forever deny your body the nutrients it needs either. This is why it is so important to head this situation off at the pass in the first place, by avoiding major binges. And if you do have one, get up the next day and get straight back on your plan.

When a client comes to my office, she may appear composed and confident. On the inside, though, most people who walk through my door are at their wits' end. They are overwhelmed with frustration and sick of trying to lose weight and failing. During their programme, I weigh them every week. I also measure body fat so I can tell them when they are putting on muscle and losing fat, even if there's no change in the number on the scales. Even so, people get incredibly discouraged when the number on the scales doesn't change or even goes up. Some people are inconsolable and, quite often, the tears just start to flow. These clients want so badly to prove that they are not a failure in my eyes and in their own hearts. The numbers on the scales seem to seal their fates as losers, but *this is simply not the case*.

There are three things you need to know here. The first is that no one is ever a loser for trying; the second is that eating healthily will feed muscle and burn fat. Some people don't immediately show weight loss because they are putting on muscle while losing body fat. Bear in mind, though, that a pound of muscle is much more attractive than a pound of fat. If you have replaced a pound of fat with a pound of muscle, you have made a big improvement in your appearance already.

The third thing to know is that you are not alone. I have been around some of the world's top fitness models and competitors, and these professionals have 'flat' weeks or 'up' weeks as well. They may lose several pounds one week, then gain back a few and at other times lose only a single pound in a week. The thing to realize is that it is a normal part of the weight loss process. Eventually the weight comes off. So don't be deceived or discouraged by the scales. And don't weigh yourself more often than once a week.

It's important to realize that the more quickly weight is lost, the more likely it is that the loss is coming from water and muscle, *not* fat. If you are losing a pound or two per week, that is actually a healthy pace. And don't forget that it is *very* hard to see weight loss on yourself, because you look at yourself in the mirror every day. Somebody who hasn't seen you for a month is likely to compliment you on your weight loss even if you can't see it yet. Don't let your own mind deceive you.

More often than not, you will notice first that your clothes fit differently and that you can once again wear the jeans and tops that have been pushed to the back of your wardrobe. There is nothing like the feeling of being able to button a button or do up a zip that wouldn't close only a few weeks earlier.

The chart below shows the progress of three women from the Skinny Chicks 10-week test group whose weight went up and back down. Each had up weeks and down weeks as well as temporary plateaus. This is a natural part of the weight loss process. Our bodies are constantly going through metabolic and hormonal changes; we shouldn't ever be discouraged by a small increase in weight.

3 TYPICAL EXAMPLES FROM SKINNY CHICKS TEST GROUP

— Hillary D. — Malinda N. — Julie H.

SKINNY CHICKS HAVE THEIR UPS AND DOWNS

Skinny Chick 10-Week Transformation

NAME: COURTNEY H.

AGE: 20

TOTAL POUNDS LOST: 15 (6.8 kg)

TOTAL INCHES LOST: 24¾ (62.9 cm)

I have been overweight all my life. My mum is big, my sister is big, my brother is big – we just have big genes. When I was at secondary school, I became very ill and I had severe stomach pains for almost a year. Eventually, I was diagnosed with Crohn's disease. Once I was put on medication, including steroids, the weight just piled on.

My dad was a single father. He was great, but he didn't have time or know how to give us the most nutritional meals. I got in the habit of eating fast foods and anything that was quick and easy, so I just kept putting on weight.

I moved to California to go to college and started to get ill again. In 2007, part of my intestine was removed. Even then, I still clung to my bad eating habits. I couldn't find a weight loss plan I could stick to or that would give me any results. I was getting depressed and desperate.

When I started the Skinny Chicks programme, I was sure it was just going to be something else I'd try for a week and then drop. But it wasn't like that at all. The programme has made me take a good look at myself and my life. I've had to face my demons and let go of things that were holding me back. Now I feel like I'm on the track to success. Christine not only taught me to eat healthily and helped me lose weight; she also made me believe that my thoughts and words become my reality.

As you can see, a small gain in a week is a normal part of every successful weight loss process. In this chart, all three women had two 'up' weeks, but eventually they lost anywhere from 11 to 20 pounds (5 to 9 kilograms).

Sometimes clients who have been through dieting extremes will put on a few pounds in the early days of starting my programme. I can recall one example of this with a very popular celebrity client whom I'll call Susan. Susan started my programme with dedication and excitement, especially when she found out that eating carbs actually helps to achieve a sleek, lean body. However, our first 2 weeks of working together were quite a challenge. Five days after starting, I received a frantic call from Susan's assistant telling me that Susan had put on 4 pounds (1.8 kilograms) and was literally freaking out because she had to be on camera that afternoon for a TV interview. This might sound like no big deal, but for a celebrity, it seemed like a career killer – something that could undermine her entire family's livelihood. I advised the assistant to keep Susan calm, and to get the wardrobe stylist to find her the nicest-looking long-sleeved shirt or jacket for the interview, as the first place her weight always showed was her arms. I also asked to see her in my office as soon as possible. When I finally met up with Susan, I could see she was retaining a lot of water – possibly a reaction to suddenly eating carbs again. Now, bear in mind that this is a beautiful and famous woman who had previously been avoiding all carbs with the exception of a sugar binge here and there. (Oh, how I understood her issues – they hit very close to home!) I had forewarned her about this, and I reminded her that for every gram of sugar the body receives, it can hold approximately 4 grams of water. Like many low-carb zealots, Susan probably thought I was full of it, but she stuck to the plan because a friend of hers had lost 16 pounds (7.3 kilograms) in 1 month on my programme. Thank goodness she did stick with it, because by the following week, the extra weight was gone and she went on to achieve dramatic results, losing a total of 7 per cent body fat in 12 weeks. Susan continues to follow my programme to this day.

So, if the scales go up a little, don't worry about it. Not only is it a natural progression, but it might even mean you're putting on muscle. Stick it out. This programme works because it's not a diet. It's the real deal for real people in real life.

CHAPTER 15

Every Day
Is a Splurge Day

What if I told you that you could be a Skinny Chick and still enjoy the foods you like and eat out without guilt? It *is* possible to strike a balance between enjoying the foods you love and living your healthiest life.

A lot of diets encourage you to have a 'splurge day' as part of the programme. Sadly, that perpetuates the attitude that a diet is a temporary restrictive programme that you can leave when you're 'done'. My response to that philosophy is: *We've been splurging our entire lives, which is how we ended up putting on weight in the first place!* Enough with the splurge days; we are real people living in a real world . . . it's time to tune in to reality. We need to pull the plug on splurge days and diets altogether.

The Skinny Chicks programme is not temporary or restrictive – it's a way of eating your whole life long so that you won't need a splurge day. Make room in your daily meals for a chocolate chip cookie once in a while or a slice of birthday cake like those sassy Skinny Chicks you know. (After all, why should they get to prance around with a dessert at a dinner party, while you sit there with a bottled water repeating, 'No thanks, I'm on a diet, I have to wait till my "splurge day".') Stop dieting, stop with the splurge days, and start living. I will cheer you on and guide you every step of the way. If a food-obsessed girl like me can actually break away from the bondage of 24-hour sugar cravings, so can you.

The Sweetest Things

By now I hope you have an understanding of the insanity that once surrounded my own eating habits. The core of that insanity was my intense love of sweets. They aren't called sweets for nothing; for me, they made my sour existence tolerable. Why? Because for a brief moment, they were the only thing that anaesthetized my sorrow. I remember talking with girlfriends literally for hours – not about guys or careers, but about *sweets!* I was never into drugs, but my cravings for sweets were so acute and powerful that I might as well have been a street addict.

Nevertheless, my addiction to sweet things was an integral part of what made me pursue a career in nutrition. And that led to this amazing discovery:

If you have a lean protein in your meal, you can choose whatever type of carbohydrate you wish.

The operative word here is *choose*. You can have *any* carbohydrate you want. That doesn't mean you can have *every* carbohydrate you want all at the same time. And most importantly, it must be part of a PC Combo. For example, if you are attending a wedding and they are serving grilled fish, green beans, roasted potatoes, bread rolls and cake, simply skip the carbs in the meal (potatoes and bread rolls – the green beans are a free food) and count a small piece of wedding cake as the carbohydrate component of your PC Combo. Just be sure to eat your dessert within 1 hour of eating your meal. You want the sugar from the dessert to be slowed down by the amino acids from the protein in the meal. All the meals in my programme are designed so that you can easily eliminate the carbs and fats and swap them for your favourite dessert.

Can you do this at every meal and still lose weight? It's possible, although I wouldn't advise it. I had a client a few years back who told me in our first appointment that she would follow my programme to the letter as long as she could eat sweets with every meal. Sounds a little strange to pay a nutritionist to help with weight loss yet demand that

The Real Skinny about Dark Chocolate

One thing some of my successful clients do is have one small piece of dark chocolate (no more than 30 grams or 1 ounce) after a healthy PC Combo meal. If you're going to choose a sweet treat, this is your best choice, as recent studies have shown that dark chocolate is actually good for your health. Dark chocolate contains flavonoids, antioxidants that help fight damage caused by free radicals. It also has heart health benefits, including helping to reduce high blood pressure and lower cholesterol. Look for dark chocolate (not milk or white chocolate) that has at least 70 per cent or higher cocoa content. Whatever your sweet preference may be, I encourage you to feel free to have the occasional treat rather than be bound to the 'diet/deprivation' mind-set. Just use your good judgment and keep eating PC Combos.

your nutritionist allow you to eat sweets. But hey, I've been there myself, so I could relate. I advised her to find low-fat sweets with fewer than 50 grams of carbohydrates, and I told her that as long as she ate them along with a lean protein, she could have her cake and eat it too! That particular client lost 25 pounds (11.3 kilograms) in 12 weeks, and even I was amazed. I don't recommend that you make this a steady habit, because obviously, sweets lack protein, fibre, vitamins, minerals and antioxidants. But that client's results show that having a dessert once in a while won't hurt or impede your progress. The Skinny Chicks programme is about living and eating in the real world.

All my clients want to find ways to get their sweets, and so do I. However, consider the following: a single piece of cheesecake from The Cheesecake Factory can have as many as 1,600 calories. A pint (568 ml) of Ben & Jerry's can easily contain more than 1,200 calories. To put that in perspective, a healthy woman weighing 9 stone 4 pounds (59 kilograms) requires around 1,500 to 1,800 calories per day to maintain her body weight. Not only that, but these desserts are extremely high in saturated fats and cholesterol. So what should a sweet-toothed Skinny Chick do?

At some point, most dieters experience a 'cave-in' and eat a huge amount of sweets after trying to deprive themselves of food for a long period. So the first thing to do is eat on a regular basis in order to stabilize your blood sugar. Once their blood sugar has been stable for 3 days or so, most of my clients find they are far less tempted to splurge.

But, if you're really desperate for that chocolate fudge cake (hey, just because I'm a nutritionist doesn't mean I don't enjoy rich desserts!), have a small serving, enjoy it, and move on. If you continue to resist, you are going to drive yourself bananas (or more likely, banana splits!)

The 100-Calorie Slippery Slope

Have you been to the supermarket lately? Next time you go, take a trip down the snack aisle. Those savvy marketers are at it again. They know we're all concerned about our weight, and they know we all still want those sweets and crisps. So what have they done? They've cleverly packaged a wide range of products, from Pringles to Jaffa Cakes, from biscuits to pretzels and nuts, in smaller 100-calorie snack packs. The idea is that because we could never buy a tube of Pringles and eat just one or two (our blood sugar levels have us on 'binge mode'), they've shrunk them into 100-calorie portions for us. Sounds like a good idea, no?

There are a number of problems with this. For one thing, you're paying top dollar for those pint-size treats. In fact, you're paying twice as much for a snack that will fill you up only half as much as a better choice, such as a piece of string cheese or some yogurt and granola.

But that's not my main problem with these tiny snacklets. If I want a piece of pecan pie for dessert, I won't be satisfied with a child-sized handful of biscuits or crisps. I'll eat the snack pack and still feel deprived. That voice inside my head will still be screaming, *I want my pecan pie!* Which means I'll probably finish off my 100-calorie treat in the blink of an eye, and before I know it, I'll have another and another . . . until I've consumed a whole meal's worth of calories. And I'll still be craving pecan pie.

So, I say, forget about the snack packs and go for the pie. Have a lean protein for dinner, have some veggies from the free food list (see Appendix), and follow it up with a small piece of the pie you've been salivating over for days. When you follow the Skinny Chicks PC Combo plan, one piece will do it for you. You will satisfy your sweet tooth without having to eat the whole pie. You won't want the whole pie because you will be eating so much and so often on this programme.

Artificial Sweeteners:
The Good, the Bad, and the Deadly!

Although it would be great if everything we ate were made of the purest, most natural ingredients, that is not always the case. For those of us watching our weight and wanting to splurge without adding extra calories, foods made with artificial sweeteners are often the answer.

They are calorie-free and they don't spike blood sugar. So what's the problem with artificial sweeteners? Well, no one is really sure, and that could be a problem. Personally, I am neutral on the subject, although I believe some sugar alternatives are better than others. It is important to consume all things in moderation. As you follow my Skinny Chicks nutrition programme, your desire for sweets will begin to diminish, and the idea of adding sweetener to your drinks and meals may lose its appeal. The great thing about this programme is that you will no longer be a slave to sugar. But I could not write a nutrition book without providing a little background information, so here's the skinny on sweeteners.

All artificial sweeteners are made of different blends of molecules that trick our tastebuds into believing that they taste something sweet. Artificial sweeteners trigger the same taste receptors as sugar does. The difference is, it only takes a tiny amount of artificial sweetener to get your tongue thinking you just consumed a large amount of sugar. Artificial sweeteners are hundreds or, in some cases, even tens of thousands of times sweeter than real sugar. For example, there are 10 teaspoons of sugar in one can of Coke, while there is less than a tenth of a teaspoon of aspartame in a Diet Coke. Because artificial sweeteners work so well in such small amounts, they add almost no calories to foods and drinks while offering the same or even a higher level of sweetness.

Although the evidence on whether artificial sweeteners are harmful to human beings is inconclusive, I strongly recommend that you use them with caution. In my experience, the overuse of artificial sweeteners can cause sugar cravings. I've witnessed clients suffering from extreme sugar cravings only to find out that they use an average of 30 to 40 packets of artificial sweetener daily. I myself can recall using 10 packets of Equal while spooning half a jar of peanut butter into my mouth.

Here are some of the most common sugar alternatives.

Aspartame: In 1996, scientists tried to link an increase in human brain cancer between the late 1970s and mid 1980s to a higher use of aspartame, but further analysis exposed inconsistencies in their data. Long-term studies on laboratory rats have found no harmful effects from the consumption of aspartame. In September 2007, a panel of 10 American researchers conducted a review of more than 500 aspartame studies and concluded that it is safe. However, if you consume moderate or large amounts of artificial sweetener, I recommend you consider the studies and decide for yourself.

Sucralose: Commonly known as Splenda. Sucralose is a sugar molecule. To create Splenda, sucralose undergoes a number of chemical alterations, including the addition of a chlorine atom. Splenda has only been on the market since 1998, thus we lack long-term studies on its side effects. The studies that have been conducted so far have failed to prove that it is harmful. David L. Katz, MD, MPH, director of the Yale Griffin Prevention Research Center in Connecticut, told the *Los Angeles Times*, 'There is no direct evidence that Splenda causes cancer. It's just a theoretical concern.' That said, I caution my clients to use any artificial sweetener, including Splenda, in moderation. And remember, a little goes a long way.

Agave nectar: This is a wonderful natural sweetener and a great alternative to artificial sweeteners in my opinion. However, agave nectar is not calorie free; it yields 20 calories per teaspoon. Agave nectar is derived from the heart of a Mexican cactus, which contains a sweet-

Skinny Chick Chat

HEY CHRISTINE! I grew up having dessert after every meal (okay, maybe not breakfast, but definitely lunch and dinner) and often sweet snacks in between. When I try to diet and cut out sweets altogether, I give up after a week or so. Can I have my sweets and diet too?

SARAH H.

SARAH: Yes you can – in moderation, of course. Just try some of the recipes beginning on page 237. If you eat out and you crave dessert, share one with your dinner companions. The caveat is that these desserts should be eaten shortly after a small, balanced meal or eaten with a lean protein. I have separated the nutrition in each meal on my programme so you can easily swap any carb and fat for a reasonable serving of your favourite dessert. Combining these tasty treats with a lean protein will help slow the speed of the sugar from these foods as its glucose molecules flow down the Blood Sugar Freeway. It is important to realize that one enormous dessert can throw off the stability of your blood sugar level for up to 3 days.

EAT WELL, CHRISTINE

sticky juice. In the 1500s, when the Spaniards arrived in Mexico, they fermented the juice of the agave plant into what we know today as tequila. More recently, agave syrup has become available in health food shops as a fantastic alternative sweetener for health-conscious individuals. The great thing about agave nectar is that it is approximately 90 per cent fructose, so it has a low glycaemic level, which, as we know, is helpful when it comes to keeping blood sugar levels steady. This makes agave a natural healthy option for people with diabetes and all people who are concerned about their waistlines. I personally use about a tablespoon of this sweetener almost every day, both in my morning tea and in my yummy Greek yogurt parfait (see the recipe on page 122).

To wrap it all up, remember that Skinny Chicks don't eat salads. They eat real foods, and they do have desserts once in a while. They don't need a separate splurge day because they eat healthily most of the time, and if they want dessert, they pair it up with a protein and eat it as part of a meal. If you build up that 'poor me, I'm so deprived' diet mind-set and never allow yourself a splurge, you're bound for a major binge. So follow the Skinny Chicks dessert guidelines and have a sweet life!

SKINNY CHICKS DESSERT GUIDELINES

1. If you're going to have dessert, have it with your meal.

2. Eat a lean protein before your dessert.

3. Swap a starchy carbohydrate from your main course for your dessert, omitting rice, potato, fruit or bread.

4. Your dessert portion should be low in fat and less than 50 grams of carbohydrates.

5. Do not have a dessert more than twice a week if you truly want to lose weight.

6. To jump-start weight loss, hold off on dessert until you've reached your goal weight.

CHAPTER 16

The Diner's Dilemma

When I was growing up and living with my grandparents, they prepared every meal at home. We had breakfast and lunch together every single day (when I was at school, Grandma packed me a sandwich), and every night at 6 p.m. there was food on the table. Sadly, cooking at home is almost a quaint notion for many people – sort of a nostalgic memory of a simpler time. Nutritionally speaking, that has been to our detriment. When you cook at home, there is no question that the food you eat is healthier and less fattening, not to mention less expensive, and it's nice to have something delicious filling the kitchen with great aromas, rather than a pile of empty takeaway containers on the worktop. As they say, 'when you cook, you're family'. That is why I have created a multitude of quick and easy meal preparations that fit into my nutrition programme nicely and, in most cases, can be prepared in less than 10 minutes.

But one thing you can be sure of is that unless you are living with your own parents or grandparents, some of your meals will come from food stands, delis, fast-food joints and restaurants. It is an inescapable fact of modern life that few of us have time to make many, much less most, of our meals at home. Therefore it is vitally important to have a plan for ordering the right food when eating out.

Restaurants want you to enjoy the taste of their food, and if that means adding a little more oil or butter, then that is what they will do. Even when you order healthy restaurant choices, you will consume more fat than you would if you prepared the same thing at home; if you choose a less healthy preparation, such as something deep-fried, who knows how much fat you are consuming? But the worst thing about eating out is that most people can't resist all the extras – a warm, soft brownie, a 'homemade' lemonade, a side of fries, a new coffee drink with whipped cream, the bread before the meal and the dessert afterwards. People who eat out often end up consuming a lot of these calorie-laden add-ons, and it can make weight control impossible. Even if you eat only one or two of these extras per week, you may sabotage your weight loss – or, even worse, put on weight.

Meet Rachelle, Who Had the Belly Fat Blues

Rachelle, a 19-year-old student, came to see me to lose the extra belly fat she had gained during her first year. She was tall, pretty, and mostly slender, but her belly area was round and protruding. I reviewed her food journal and noticed that she and her friends ate at a restaurant every night. They would always start with bread and butter, maybe some tortilla chips and salsa, or sometimes potato skins or mozzarella cheese sticks. She didn't want to say no when her friends were eating, so she ate along with them. She told me that since she was eating all the extra stuff, she usually just ordered a salad for dinner (and we know how that works). When dessert time rolled around, they would share one between them. All these little extras had the not surprising effect of saddling Rachelle with the extra pounds she did not want.

When I explained to Rachelle about blood sugar and the PC Combo, she said, 'Wow, that's all I have to do? I'll try it.' She took the info and ran with it. In 10 weeks, she lost 14 pounds (6.4 kilograms) and looked fantastic. She was overflowing with confidence and personality. Now, when she met up with friends for dinner, she no longer felt out of control, so she could easily say no to the mozzarella stick and nacho appetizers. When she'd order a substantial main course, her friends would pepper her with questions about how she could eat the meals she was eating and still lose

Skinny Chick 10-Week Transformation

NAME: JENNIFER K.

AGE: 37

TOTAL POUNDS LOST: 21 (9.5 kg)

TOTAL INCHES LOST: 22 (55.9 cm)

In my mind, I have been overweight all my life. As an adult, I'm finally realizing that the childhood image I've always held of myself (the fat girl) is untrue. Yes, I carried a few extra pounds, as a young girl rarely made good food choices and spent more time reading or watching TV than recommended, but I didn't become truly obese until after secondary school.

One of my earliest memories is of a relative making me a breakfast different from my brother's because 'it was time for me to lose some weight'. I can remember being surprised and actually thinking, *When did it go from baby fat to just fat?* I was 7 or 8 years old. So I struggled.

After school, I embarked on a low-fat diet. I counted fat grams and did lose inches and weight – but I gained it back. At 25 years old, after a major break-up, I finally did it right. I ate healthy meals prepared at home, exercised regularly and enjoyed once-monthly 'cheat weekends', where pizza and brownies were meals of choice. That lasted 5 months, but when I moved in with roommates, I reverted to the old habits. I was self-conscious about exercising where people could see me, and I ate what they cooked rather than rocking the boat.

Today, I make better choices more often, but for the most part, this has only stopped the weight gain rather than inducing weight loss. I am still rather inactive, and my old friends, books and TV, are never far away.

The best thing about the Skinny Chicks programme is that my whole outlook on life has changed since I started. I am working to alter my relationship with food, and this plan has allowed me to really define and enjoy the healthy foods available to me. I certainly have noticed that my body is changing. Both my stomach and my bottom have become smaller. I have much more energy, which allows me to participate in many more things than I was previously doing. I believe I am making much better choices for myself, and I definitely plan to stick with this programme for the long haul.

Since I started the programme, I eat more often than I used to. I take supplements. I am aware of the best options for me, and I don't have to have a meal loaded with unhealthy carbs in order to enjoy what I'm eating. I now look forward to a meal that not only tastes good, but that also has nutritional value as well.

weight. She had to tell them that her foods were actually a lot healthier than their salads. Ten weeks, a flat tummy and 14 pounds (6.4 kilograms) later, her friends were convinced.

Your Best Bets Eating Out

Once you've got a handle on all those diet-busting extras, the next thing to do is figure out what in the world to order. Don't worry; no matter where you choose to dine, I guarantee you can find great healthy choices to keep you on your plan. I have designed meal plans that include favourite restaurants for more than 1,000 of my clients. Here are some helpful examples:

- **Food stands:** Many of our meals come from a cafeteria at work, a food court at the shopping mall, or some other food stand-type location. What can you order from these places and stay on your food plan? I always look for a selection that contains a nice helping of chicken breast, turkey or fish along with a healthy carb. Examples: chicken or fish soft tacos, deli turkey sandwiches, tomato-based pasta with chicken, chicken burritos (hold the soured cream and cheese), chicken teriyaki with rice, turkey burgers on a wholemeal bun and grilled chicken/salmon/tuna sandwiches. If there is too much sauce, butter, mayonnaise or cheese on your food, just scrape some of it off. Every little bit of these high-fat items makes a big difference. (You can use all the ketchup, mustard and salsa you want.) The things to avoid are your standard fare: hot dogs, sausages, hamburgers, chips, nachos, milkshakes, Danish pastries, doughnuts and ice cream. Avoid any fried foods, cream sauces and regular fizzy drinks.

- **Delis:** Delis are a great place to grab a healthy bite. Order a smoked turkey, chicken breast or lean ham sandwich with no cheese and light mayo, then pile on the vegetables and salad to your heart's content. The things to avoid are tuna salad or chicken salad sandwiches, salami and processed meats and regular cheese.

- **Casual restaurants/diners/takeaway:** Again, I recommend looking for dishes that are based on chicken, turkey or fish and sometimes lean steak (preferably filet mignon, if you can afford it). Here is a partial list of my favourites:

  - **Asian:** Chicken stir-fry or chicken teriyaki plus a side salad; hold the dressing and use rice vinegar
  - **Diner:** Roasted turkey breast with a baked potato, hold the mash
  - **Greek:** Chicken skewers with rice; hold the hummus
  - **Grill:** Grilled fish with rice and veggies; hold the oil; use lemon and herbs for seasoning
  - **Indian:** Chicken tikka with rice and veggies; hold the masala cream sauce
  - **Italian:** Pasta with tomato sauce with chicken or prawns, plus a side salad (use balsamic vinegar instead of dressing); hold the cheese and cream sauces
  - **Mexican:** Grilled chicken or shrimp fajitas or tacos; hold the guacamole, cheese and soured cream
  - **Thai:** Garlic chicken with rice and steamed veggies

  This list could go on and on, but I think you get the idea. You'll find that healthy choices are available no matter what type of restaurant you frequent, if you are vigilant about holding the high-fat extras like cheese and soured cream.

  Look for the dishes that are based on healthy lean proteins. What should you avoid? As we know, those speciality salads tend to be extremely high in calories and fat. Anything with a creamy sauce is going to be overloaded with fat (fettuccine Alfredo would be enemy number one). Anything involving cheese, soured cream, butter or lots of oil (such as deep-fried foods) is definitely on the 'best to avoid' list. Remember that cheese, soured cream and butter are animal-based high-fat foods whose fat is mostly saturated. Many, many dishes combine multiple high-fat offenders – like deep-fried mozzarella sticks dipped in ranch dressing, or deep-fried fish tacos with soured cream. As you start to recognize the primary high-fat food sources, it becomes easier to find healthy choices in your own life.

- **Fine dining:** When dining in a full-service restaurant, my best advice is that you eat a small meal 2 hours before your reservation. Often you end up sitting down an hour late for various reasons, and you don't want to be starving. Try not to eat the bread before dinner. This isn't always easy to do when you sit down to eat and you are so hungry that you're ready to gnaw on your own arm. But bread on an empty stomach causes a rapid rise in blood sugar. Better to order a chicken skewer or a crab or prawn cocktail (i.e. something that is primarily protein) as an appetizer straight away and ask the waiter take the bread back to where it came from.

  When you do order your main course, again stay away from the high-fat foods: cream sauces, cheesy dishes, fried foods and oily or buttery dishes. Stay with tomato-based sauces and grilled meat cuts such as fish, chicken and filet mignon.

  For all of my specifics, refer to the meal plans found in Chapter 11, which include healthy choices from many favourite restaurants. Additionally, I have created a 'fast-food guide' at www.christineavanti.com for inquiring minds who want to know the best and worst fast-food eats. I recommend you check it out if you are not able to prepare your own meals on a regular basis. I'm not a fan of fast food, but I realize that in today's world, the reality is most people end up eating at fast-food restaurants more often than they plan to, so it's best to be prepared.

CHAPTER 17

Skinny Chicks Helpful Tricks

Life isn't perfect. That's one of the things that makes 'dieting' so hard. I'm asking you to make changes in your lifestyle: to eat every 4 hours, to combine carbs and proteins and to exercise five times a week. If you are able to do all those things all the time, more power to you. If you can't, all it means is that you're a human being. If you can't always follow the plan perfectly every time, don't worry; it's not the end of the world. If perfection were the only goal, few people would make it past the second day. Don't cave in and have a huge binge; just get right back on your plan.

Fortunately, there are lots of options for keeping your weight loss going even when the unexpected occurs. This chapter will help you cope when that happens.

Timing Is Everything

What if you can't eat on the 4-hour mark? What if you're invited to a fabulous party where everyone will be eating all kinds of food for 5 straight hours? What if you were stuck at work and couldn't eat for 8 hours – and then ate a whole bag of Kettle Chips? What if it is a holiday or somebody's birthday? What if your life is not regimented with military precision?

Most of us do not run our lives with military precision, and we really wouldn't want to. With some foresight and planning, though, you can still fit in the meals you need to keep your brain supplied with glucose and thus keep your body lean and mean. Let's say your plan calls for you to eat at 8 a.m., 12 p.m. and 4 p.m., but you are invited to a dinner party at 6 p.m. Rather than starve yourself until 6 (and more than likely overeat at dinner), just cut your 4 p.m. meal in half, then go and have dinner at 6 p.m. (I recommend that you have a half-meal here, unless you are tremendously hungry; in that case, have a full meal and wait 4 hours until your next meal if you are still awake at that time.) As long as you eat the proper balance of nutrients at every meal, you will be fine. You may actually have as many as six small meals in a given day. As long as you keep them balanced and modestly portioned, you'll be sticking to your plan. In fact, this is very similar to the way professional athletes and celebrities eat.

Let's look at some specific situations and strategies for coping with them.

The Mega-Binge Disaster: Social Obligations

What if you find yourself at a huge dinner party where you are served seven courses? Many of my socially active clients have this dilemma. In 2004, I began working with a client by the name of Kallissa. Kallissa started the Skinny Chicks programme at 28 per cent body fat and ended at 19 per cent, and she has been able to maintain her results for more than 3 years despite her very busy work and social schedule. Here is Kallissa's story.

Kallissa was an avid exerciser and healthy eater for many years, but her career as an executive producer of three hit shows on MTV made it nearly impossible for her to stick to her goals. Kallissa had a staff of more than 150 people, and to reward their hard work, Kallissa liked to throw fun events for holidays and premieres, and wrap parties. This added up to two or three major parties each month, and that did not include the other social commitments that come with the territory of being a Hollywood producer. With a schedule like Kallissa's, you'd think it would be almost impossible to adhere to my Skinny Chicks nutrition plan. Kallissa asked me for tips on how to navigate her way through these events so that she could continue on the plan in a way that would not be obvious to onlookers.

Here are some of the tips I gave her:

- **Never go to an event on an empty stomach.** Kallissa often ate light cheese strings and a small piece of fruit in the car or taxi on her way to an event or hot spot.

- **Nurse one drink all night** (see page 278 for low-calorie drinks). When Kallissa arrived at a function, she would order a small glass of champagne (approximately 150 ml/¼ pint) and sip on this 100-calorie drink for an hour or even 2 hours, during which time her colleagues might have had three or four drinks.

- **Order food before you start drinking.** If you're going to a bar or restaurant where food is served, eat first, *then* drink. If you start with alcohol, you're more likely to give in to temptation and have something outside your plan. I advised Kallissa to order a lean protein prepared with very little oil and some high-fibre carbohydrates such as brown rice or steamed veggies. Kallissa's favourite 'bar' meal was prawn cocktail, one or two bites of another appetizer if one was ordered by someone in her party and one small glass of champagne.

- **Don't punish yourself for slipping up.** I usually tell my clients to try to avoid challenging social situations for the first 10 weeks of the Skinny Chicks programme, but I know that's not always possible. If you do go out and you do slip up, don't starve yourself the next day. Simply go right back to your plan. Weight loss, like life, doesn't go in a straight line; there are ups and downs. If you go right back to your plan, your weight will continue to drop.

Anticipate Starvation Solutions

What if you are stuck on the road or at work and can't take a break to eat? What if you are in an important meeting and eating is out of the question? These are the toughest situations and the ones I find the toughest to deal with. My office gets so busy at times that my scheduled meal breaks get absorbed if a client turns up late, or an appointment goes past its allotted 30 minutes. When I miss an appointed meal time by an hour, two or even more, I start to feel a little loopy. At times like these, making good food choices is almost impossible. Often, I am so short of time that I only have 5 minutes to run down and grab something from the Starbucks coffee bar in my building. By that time, I'm starving and feel tempted to order the chocolate muffin and a double mocha. I have to remind myself to take a deep breath and calm down. I tell myself, 'Look. You're hungry and your blood sugar is low. Just stick to the plan and you'll be fine.' Then I order a turkey sandwich and fruit salad . . . and I feel more energized than if I had had the double mocha and muffin.

The key is to *anticipate* these situations and eat before they happen. Keep a high-fibre protein bar in your handbag, briefcase or car. I don't recommend these as meal replacements, and they may contain additives I'd rather avoid, but at a pinch they are far better than a pastry or greasy fast food. If you're stuck in a long meeting, use the tea breaks to eat a quick, healthy bite and keep your blood sugar on an even keel. That's the best way to stay sharp – and on your plan.

Be Efficient

One great strategy to help avoid missing meals is to cook or buy more than one meal at a time. Your life is busy; why should you spend more time than you have to shopping, preparing and clearing up? If you are going to cook, make enough for two or three meals so you can have leftovers. The same goes for ordering takeaways or eating out. This way, you are unlikely to overeat and you'll already have one of tomorrow's meals ready to go. This is also a great help when you feel hungry and you want something to eat *right now*. If you have leftovers readily available, you're less likely to veer off your plan.

Meet Dr John, the Coke Fiend

One of my clients, John, was an ophthalmologist. He was in his sixties and appeared to be in decent shape; he was tall and thin. He had been referred to me by his own doctor after an annual check-up. Despite his mostly healthy appearance, his blood tests showed that he was border-line diabetic, so his doctor recommended that I review his diet.

I reviewed his food journal and discovered that he ate nothing all day long, then had a large dinner at night. The only thing that kept him going during the day was quaffing a Coke whenever he had a break. With each Coke, John's body would receive a massive infusion of sugar.

John said, 'I don't have time to eat. I see patients all day long. In between patients, I drink Coca-Cola and that's all the time I've got. Besides that, I love drinking Coke, so don't tell me to quit.'

I told him he had to start eating breakfast every day and get his secretaries to schedule time between patients for lunch and one mid-afternoon meal. Now, bear in mind, this is a successful medical professional who was not overweight. When I laid out his meal plans and showed him that they did not include Cokes, he was impatient and very annoyed.

'Oh c'mon, there's got to be something else. Can't you give me a supplement or some kind of drink? You can't be serious. How can I eat real food all day long? Why should I pay you to tell me to give up my Cokes? I am *not* giving up my Cokes, and I also like having a dessert at night.' The concept of eating real food during the day seemed inconve-nient and as foreign to John as reading Chinese. Cokes, on the other hand, were easy and readily available.

At this point, I got dead serious with John. 'Do you have a family?' I asked.

'Yes.'

'Do you have children?'

'Yes.'

'Do you have grandchildren?'

'Yes.'

'Do you want to see them grow up?'

'Well, of course!'

'Then you are going to have to start eating real food and stabilizing your blood sugar or you won't. You are pre-diabetic and, being a medical person, you should know what happens to diabetic people who do not eat properly. They can end up on dialysis, go blind, lose extremities to amputation and eventually die from their condition.' For some reason it hadn't occurred to John that his all-cola diet was literally ushering him to an early grave. Reluctantly, he decided to try my plan. He started eating breakfast and quick but balanced meals twice a day between patients. Although weight loss was not his goal, he ended up losing 10 pounds (4.5 kilograms) and reducing his body fat by 3 per cent by the 10th week of my programme.

More importantly, 2 months later, a blood test showed that John was no longer pre-diabetic. He was in much brighter spirits and had more energy. He smiled as he told me that his secretaries said he had been a much nicer person over the past 2 months. The unstable blood sugar levels had been causing his moods to go haywire. John's 30-year habit had seemed to work for him, but inside, his body was calling out for a change. The happy result? John has put his life back on a healthy track, he has avoided diabetes, and he has made life better for all the people around him.

PART V

SKINNY CHICKS

GET IN

THE KITCHEN

Recipes

In this section, you'll find recipes for all the dishes mentioned in the meal plans on pages 122 to 165, plus extra breakfast, lunch, dinner, and dessert recipes for planning your own menus.

By now I hope you have realized that it's not just how *much* you eat but what you eat that matters. Of course, you could satisfy your body's need for fuel – and probably come up with perfectly adequate PC combos – by defrosting a frozen meal every day. But choosing top-quality ingredients and preparing them with care will result in meals that satisfy so much more than just your basic physiological needs.

As a child, I often spent weekends with my grandparents on their farm. In the morning, I was up early to pick fruit and vegetables with Grandpa Luigi for the big Sunday afternoon feast – a tradition we never missed. My entire family – grandparents, aunts, uncles, cousins, my mum, my two sisters and me – gathered around the table to eat a wonderful meal cooked with love by my grandmother. As we walked around the farm, Grandpa taught me about growing and caring for the fruits, vegetables and herbs – and about life.

Anybody who has ever eaten fresh farm-grown produce knows how much better it tastes than commercially grown products. From the fresh salad to the homemade pasta to the local meat to the homemade wine, the whole meal was balanced, home-grown and homemade, with plenty of variety.

Long before fad dieting ever started, Grandma and Grandpa were eating healthy, natural, nutritious meals from the earth that included protein, carbohydrates and fats. Sometimes in my research I can hear Grandpa Luigi saying, 'Chris, a gooda meal is like a gooda lifa – needs a gooda balance.'

When Grandpa Luigi passed away, his strength helped me through the tough times before I finally found my calling as a nutritionist. Today,

I think of him with every meal I make. Most importantly, I feel empowered by something Grandpa Luigi knew all along – that food is meant to be a joyful part of life that brings people together. Slowly and surely, as the Skinny Chicks programme came together, the depressed, hopeless feelings of futility so familiar to dieters were replaced by feelings of health and confidence, as the way I eat was changed for ever.

These are the recipes that I've shared with my clients and that I prepare nightly for myself and my husband. Paired with the grab-and-go suggestions you'll find in the meal plans, they keep us satisfied, well nourished and happy at the table. I hope you will enjoy these recipes and be inspired to adapt some of your favourite recipes to PC combos, too!

Christine's High-Protein Pumpkin Ginger Pancakes

Nutrition facts per serving: 376 calories, 21 g protein,
53 g carbohydrates, 10 g fat SERVES 4 (2 PANCAKES PER SERVING)

145 g (5 oz) wholemeal flour

2 tbsp brown sugar

1 tsp baking powder

½ tsp bicarbonate of soda

½ tsp cinnamon

½ tsp ginger

¼ tsp salt

240 ml (8 fl oz) light vanilla soya milk

2 scoops protein powder
(any brand that yields
20 g protein per scoop)

150 g (5½ oz) low-fat Greek-style
vanilla yogurt

12 tbsp canned pumpkin

2 extra-large egg whites

2 tbsp butter,
slightly melted

2 slices crystallized ginger, diced

2 tbsp cold butter

Non-stick cooking spray

4 tbsp maple syrup

In a large mixing bowl, combine the first 7 ingredients and set aside.

In a blender, combine the soya milk and protein powder and blend for
30 seconds, then pour into a medium bowl. To the protein mixture, add the
yogurt, pumpkin, egg whites and butter, and mix well.

Add the liquid mixture to the dry ingredients and stir just until moist.
Do not overmix the pancake batter.

Warm a large frying pan over medium-low heat. Meanwhile, add the ginger
to the butter, mix well and set aside.

Spray the frying pan with cooking spray. Ladle the pancake batter into the
frying pan, using 60 ml (2 fl oz) of batter for each pancake. Let each pancake
cook for 2 to 3 minutes per side. Spread lightly with ginger butter and ½ tbsp
of syrup per pancake.

PROTEIN POWERED	CARBOHYDRATE CONCENTRATED	FAT FRIENDLY	FREE FOODS
Protein powder, egg whites, low-fat Greek yogurt	Wholemeal flour, sugar, soya milk, pumpkin, crystallized ginger, maple syrup	Butter, cooking spray	Baking powder, bicarbonate of soda, cinnamon, ginger

Blueberry Blinis

Nutrition facts per serving: 391 calories, 28 g protein,
56 g carbohydrates, 6 g fat SERVES 4 (3 BLINIS PER SERVING)

350 g (12½ oz) low-fat cottage cheese

230 g (8 oz) extra light cream cheese

120 ml (4 fl oz) liquid egg white

75 g (2½ oz) blueberry conserve

1 tbsp lemon juice

Non-stick cooking spray

12 shop-bought crepes

115 g (4 oz) fresh blueberries

Preheat the oven to 180ºC/350ºF/gas 4.

Mix the first 5 ingredients together in a bowl until well combined.

Spray a large baking tray with cooking spray.

Place 2 crepes flat on to the baking tray, and put one-twelfth of the cheese mixture into the middle of each crepe.

Shape the crepe into a rectangle by loosely folding in the short ends of the crepe first, and then each of the sides.

Repeat for the remaining crepes.

Bake for 12 to 15 minutes, or until golden brown.

Top with the fresh blueberries.

PROTEIN POWERED	CARBOHYDRATE CONCENTRATED	FAT FRIENDLY	FREE FOODS
Cottage cheese, cream cheese, egg whites	Blueberry conserve, crepes, blueberries	Cooking spray	Lemon juice

Nutrition facts calculated by Menu Magic Personal Chef Software, Version 2.6, 2008, Kreotek, LLC, Rio Rancho, New Mexico.

CHRISTINE'S NUTRITION NUGGETS Blueberries are one of the highest antioxidant-loaded fruits, and they contain pectin, a good fibre that binds to toxins. They also contain a compound, epicatechin, similar to that found in cranberries, that helps prevent urinary tract infections.

Breakfast Bagel Sandwich

Nutrition facts per serving: 369 calories, 27 g protein,
44 g carbohydrates, 9 g fat SERVES 1

. . . .

1 wholemeal or multigrain bagel

Non-stick cooking spray

1 slice Canadian bacon

1 tsp omega-3 spread

120 ml (4 fl oz) liquid egg white

1 pinch each of salt and ground black pepper

2 tbsp light cream cheese

1 small tomato, sliced

Toast the bagel and set aside.

Coat a non-stick pan with cooking spray and cook the Canadian bacon over a medium–low heat.

When the bacon is cooked, remove it from the pan and set aside. Add the omega-3 spread to the pan.

Pour in the egg whites and sprinkle with the salt and pepper. While the egg is setting, chop the bacon.

When most of the egg is set, use a spatula to loosen the egg from the pan, allowing any uncooked egg to run off into the pan.

Sprinkle the chopped bacon onto the egg while it's still wet. Then fold in the sides of the egg to make a square. Flip the egg square to finish cooking.

Spread the cream cheese onto the bagel.

When the egg is firm, place it on the bagel, add the tomato and serve.

PROTEIN POWERED	CARBOHYDRATE CONCENTRATED	FAT FRIENDLY	FREE FOODS
Canadian bacon, egg whites, cream cheese	Bagel	Cooking spray, omega-3 spread	Tomato

 CHRISTINE'S NUTRITION NUGGETS Tomatoes have plenty of immune-boosting vitamin C, blood pressure-lowering potassium and potential cancer-fighting flavonoids.

Cinnamon Raisin Oaty Muffins

Nutrition facts per serving: 394 calories, 25 g protein,
54 g carbohydrates, 9 g fat SERVES 4 (3 MUFFINS PER SERVING)
• •

Non-stick cooking spray
320 ml (11 fl oz) liquid egg white
250 g (9 oz) low-fat cottage cheese
60 g (2 oz) omega-3 spread
125 g (4½ oz) porridge oats
125 g (4½ oz) raisins, chopped
3 tbsp cinnamon
2 tsp agave nectar
3 tbsp vanilla-flavoured egg white protein powder

Preheat the oven to 180ºC/350ºF/gas 4.

Spray a 12-cup muffin tin with cooking spray.

In a large bowl, mix the egg whites, cottage cheese and omega-3 spread until thoroughly combined.

Add the porridge oats and mix well. Stir in the remaining ingredients.

Divide the batter among the prepared muffin cups.

Bake for 25 to 30 minutes. The muffins are done when a toothpick inserted into the centre of a muffin comes out clean.

PROTEIN POWERED	CARBOHYDRATE CONCENTRATED	FAT FRIENDLY	FREE FOODS
Egg whites, cottage cheese, protein powder	Oats, raisins	Cooking spray, omega-3 spread	Cinnamon, agave nectar

CHRISTINE'S NUTRITION NUGGETS Egg whites are an excellent source of protein, amino acids, zinc, and B vitamins.

Berry Good Stuffed French Toast

Nutrition facts per serving: 390 calories, 23 g protein,
53 g carbohydrates, 8 g fat SERVES 1

- -

2 tbsp low-sugar raspberry spread

1 tbsp fresh raspberries

2 tbsp light cream cheese

2 large slices wholemeal bread

120 ml (4 fl oz) liquid egg whites

Non-stick cooking spray

1 mint leaf

In a small bowl, mix the raspberry spread, raspberries and cream cheese together until smooth.

Spread the mixture onto one side of one slice of bread and cover with the other slice to make a sandwich.

Pour the egg whites into a bowl. Dip and soak both sides of the sandwich in the eggs.

Coat a non-stick pan with cooking spray and warm over medium heat.

Cook the sandwich on each side for approximately 2 to 3 minutes, or until the egg is cooked and the sandwich is golden brown.

Garnish with the mint leaf.

PROTEIN POWERED	CARBOHYDRATE CONCENTRATED	FAT FRIENDLY	FREE FOODS
Light cream cheese, egg whites	Raspberry spread, fresh raspberries, wholemeal bread	Cooking spray	Mint leaf

Nutrition facts calculated by Menu Magic Personal Chef Software, Version 2.6, 2008, Kreotek, LLC, Rio Rancho, New Mexico.

Asian Chicken Salad

Nutrition facts per serving: 335 calories, 28 g protein,
42 g carbohydrates, 8 g fat SERVES 2
· ·

SALAD

2 medium chicken breasts,
grilled and diced

450 g (1 lb) romaine lettuce,
inner leaves

60 g (2 oz) sugar snap peas

½ red pepper, cut into rings

75 g (2½ oz) shredded cabbage

1 tbsp chopped coriander

2 tbsp Christine's Asian Fusion
Dressing

135 g (4¾ oz) steamed brown rice

CHRISTINE'S ASIAN FUSION DRESSING

2 tsp sesame oil

1 tsp sesame seeds, toasted

¼ tsp brown sugar

1 tbsp rice vinegar

1 tbsp soy sauce

1 tsp fresh lime juice

1 tsp water

TO MAKE THE SALAD:
Combine the first 6 ingredients in a large bowl and serve with the Asian
dressing and rice on the side.

TO MAKE THE DRESSING:
Combine all of the ingredients in a small bowl and whisk for 30 seconds.

PROTEIN POWERED	CARBOHYDRATE CONCENTRATED	FAT FRIENDLY	FREE FOODS
Chicken breast	Sugar snap peas, brown rice	Asian fusion dressing	Romaine lettuce, red pepper, cabbage, coriander

CHRISTINE'S NUTRITION NUGGETS Skinny chicks don't eat fattening salads, but they sure can enjoy a crisp and bountiful salad, loaded with healthy vegetables and a low-cal dressing. Just don't forget to have it with a healthy carb so that your blood sugar doesn't stay low, causing you to crave sugar a few hours later.

Thai Chicken Lettuce Cups

Nutrition facts per serving: 393 calories, 28 g protein,
49 g carbohydrates, 9 g fat SERVES 4

· ·

60 ml (2 fl oz) lime juice

120 ml (4 fl oz) light coconut milk

2 tbsp peanut butter

1 tsp crushed chillies

285 g (10 oz) cooked boneless,
skinless chicken breasts, chopped

250 g (9 oz) cooked brown rice

12 butterhead lettuce or romaine
leaves

225 g (8 oz) carrot, grated

½ medium cucumber, sliced

300 g (10½ oz) mandarin oranges

3 spring onions, chopped

2 tbsp fresh coriander, chopped

In a large bowl, mix the first 4 ingredients together until smooth.

Stir in the chicken and rice until well coated.

Divide the mixture into 12 piles and fill the lettuce leaves.

Add the remaining ingredients evenly on top of the lettuce cups.

PROTEIN POWERED	CARBOHYDRATE CONCENTRATED	FAT FRIENDLY	FREE FOODS
Chicken breast	Brown rice, carrot, mandarin oranges	Coconut milk, peanut butter	Lime juice, crushed chillies, romaine, cucumber, spring onions, coriander

CHRISTINE'S NUTRITION NUGGETS Mandarin oranges and carrots have high amounts of vitamin C, which has been shown in research studies to prevent stress-related weight gain, particularly in the belly.

Guiltless Turkey Nachos

Nutrition facts per serving: 381 calories, 28 g protein,
45 g carbohydrates, 10 g fat SERVES 4

3 large wholewheat tortillas

350 g (12 oz) tinned pinto beans,
rinsed and drained

Non-stick cooking spray

285 g (10 oz) lean turkey mince

2 tsp taco seasoning

115 g (4 oz) chopped tomatoes

40 g (1¼ oz) low-fat, hard cheese,
grated

4 tbsp jalapeño chilli peppers, from
a jar, diced

3 spring onions, chopped

2 tbsp fresh coriander, chopped

Preheat the oven to 190ºC/375ºF/gas 5.

Cut each tortilla into 16 chip-size pieces. Spread the pieces out on a baking
sheet and cook for 10 minutes or until crisp.

Transfer the chips to an ovenproof serving dish and spread the beans evenly
on top.

In a frying pan coated with cooking spray, cook the turkey with the taco
seasoning over medium-high heat.

When the turkey is just slightly pink, add the tomatoes and reduce the heat
to simmer. Simmer for approximately 5 minutes, or until the turkey is fully
cooked and any liquid is cooked off.

Spread the turkey over the beans and chips. Sprinkle on the remaining
ingredients in the order listed.

Bake for approximately 5 minutes, or until the cheese is melted.

PROTEIN POWERED	CARBOHYDRATE CONCENTRATED	FAT FRIENDLY	FREE FOODS
Lean turkey mince, low-fat cheese	Wholewheat tortillas, pinto beans, chopped tomatoes	Cooking spray	Taco seasoning, jalapeño chilli pepper, spring onions, coriander

*Nutrition facts calculated by Menu Magic Personal Chef Software, Version 2.6, 2008,
Kreotek, LLC, Rio Rancho, New Mexico.*

CHRISTINE'S NUTRITION NUGGETS Pinto beans are a good source of iron, with 2 milligrams
per ½-cup serving.

Sicilian Chicken Soup

Nutrition facts per serving: 390 calories, 26 g protein,
51 g carbohydrates, 7 g fat SERVES 8

· ·

450 g (16 oz) boneless, skinless chicken breasts

Extra virgin olive oil spray

2 cloves garlic, finely chopped

¼ tsp cayenne pepper

1 tsp crushed chillies

1 tsp garlic salt

350 ml (12 fl oz) water

2 litres (3½ pints) low-salt chicken stock

8 sticks celery, diced

230 g (8 oz) baby carrots, diced

1 onion, diced

100 g (3½ oz) wholemeal orzo pasta

3 tbsp pesto, from a jar

4 tbsp fresh lemon juice

½ tsp salt

1 tsp ground black pepper

60 g (2 oz) Parmesan cheese, grated

16 slices wholemeal sourdough bread, toasted

Wash and pat dry the chicken, then cut into small cubes. Place in a large bowl and coat with olive oil spray. Add the next 4 ingredients and mix together so that the spices evenly coat the chicken. Set aside.

Bring the water and chicken stock to the boil in a large pan. Stir in the celery, carrots and onion and bring to the boil. Cook for 10 minutes. Add the chicken and continue to boil for 5 minutes. Add the orzo and boil for 4 more minutes, or until the chicken is cooked through. Turn off the heat, add the pesto, lemon juice, salt and pepper, and stir well. Finally add the Parmesan; stir again.

Serve with 2 slices of toast per serving.

PROTEIN POWERED	CARBOHYDRATE CONCENTRATED	FAT FRIENDLY	FREE FOODS
Chicken, Parmesan cheese	Carrots, wholemeal orzo pasta, wholemeal sourdough bread	Extra virgin olive oil, pesto	Herbs, spices, chicken stock, celery, onion, lemon juice

CHRISTINE'S NUTRITION NUGGETS The carrots in this soup provide high amounts of vitamin A (in the form of beta-carotene). Research suggests that vitamin A helps to protect skin and extends its youthful appearance.

Grilled Low-Fat Cheese Sandwich

Nutrition facts per serving: 335 calories, 24 g protein,
48 g carbohydrates, 5 g fat SERVES 1
• •

1½ slices low-fat Swiss-style cheese
2 large slices wholemeal bread
1 small tomato, sliced
¼ tsp dried oregano
1½ slices low-fat Cheddar cheese
2 tsp omega-3 spread

Place the Swiss-style cheese on one side of a slice of bread. Then place the tomato slices on top and sprinkle with the oregano.

Follow with the Cheddar and the second piece of bread.

Melt the omega-3 spread in a frying pan over medium heat and cook the sandwich for 1 to 2 minutes on each side, or until the cheese is melted and the bread is toasty.

PROTEIN POWERED	CARBOHYDRATE CONCENTRATED	FAT FRIENDLY	FREE FOODS
Low-fat Swiss cheese, low-fat Cheddar cheese	Wholemeal bread	Omega-3 spread	Tomato, dried oregano

Nutrition facts calculated by Menu Magic Personal Chef Software, Version 2.6, 2008, Kreotek, LLC, Rio Rancho, New Mexico.

CHRISTINE'S NUTRITION NUGGETS Low-fat cheese is a far better option than full-fat cheese. When shopping for cheese, read the nutrition facts labels and you will notice that full-fat cheese has the same amount of fat as it does protein per serving (and sometimes more!). Full-fat cheese is also high in saturated fats, which are associated with heart disease.

Bruschetta Chicken Wrap

Nutrition facts per serving: 367 calories, 27 g protein,
46 g carbohydrates, 8 g fat SERVES 1

• •

1 medium tomato, chopped

1 tbsp chopped fresh basil

1 tsp garlic, finely chopped

2 tbsp low-fat balsamic dressing

½ tsp extra virgin olive oil

60 g (2 oz) cooked boneless, skinless chicken breast, thinly sliced

30 g (1 oz) fresh spinach

1 large wholewheat tortilla

In a medium bowl, toss the first 7 ingredients together.

Place the mixture in the centre of the tortilla. Fold the bottom side in and then fold in the sides.

PROTEIN POWERED	CARBOHYDRATE CONCENTRATED	FAT FRIENDLY	FREE FOODS
Chicken breast	Wholewheat tortilla	Extra virgin olive oil	Tomato, basil, garlic, low-fat dressing, spinach

Nutrition facts calculated by Menu Magic Personal Chef Software, Version 2.6, 2008, Kreotek, LLC, Rio Rancho, New Mexico.

CHRISTINE'S NUTRITION NUGGETS Garlic contains a phytonutrient called allicin, which is known to destroy bad bacteria such as yeast and fungi in the intestines.

No-Fry Chicken Fried Rice

Nutrition facts per serving: 381 calories, 28 g protein,
45 g carbohydrates, 10 g fat SERVES 4
· ·

60 ml (2 fl oz) low-sodium soy sauce

1 tbsp oyster sauce

1 tbsp grated ginger

1 tbsp garlic, finely chopped

120 ml (4 fl oz) low-salt
chicken stock

2 tsp extra virgin olive oil

1 tsp omega-3 spread

75 g (2½ oz) chopped red cabbage

450 g (1 lb) broccoli florets, cut
small

1 chopped red pepper

90 g (3 oz) chopped spring onions

400 g (14 oz) brown rice, cooked

285 g (10 oz) boneless, skinless
chicken breasts, grilled and chopped

2 tbsp toasted sesame seeds

1 tsp crushed chillies

In a small bowl, mix together the soy sauce, oyster sauce, ginger, garlic and chicken stock and set aside.

In a large wok or frying pan, heat the oil and omega-3 spread over medium-high heat. Sauté the vegetables for approximately 2 minutes.

Add the soy mixture, then add the rice and mix well.

When the rice is almost heated, add the chicken and cook until heated through, approximately 3 to 5 minutes.

Transfer to a serving dish and sprinkle with the sesame seeds and crushed chillies.

PROTEIN POWERED	CARBOHYDRATE CONCENTRATED	FAT FRIENDLY	FREE FOODS
Chicken breast	Brown rice	Extra virgin olive oil	Soy sauce, oyster sauce, ginger, chicken stock, red cabbage, broccoli, red pepper, spring onions, crushed chillies

Nutrition facts calculated by Menu Magic Personal Chef Software, Version 2.6, 2008, Kreotek, LLC, Rio Rancho, New Mexico.

CHRISTINE'S NUTRITION NUGGETS Stir-frying vegetables causes fewer vitamins to be lost than boiling them does. Ginger is an ancient Chinese cure for colds. Fresh ginger might fight viruses by causing the body to sweat out toxins.

Christine's Pasta and Spicy Red Sauce

Nutrition facts per serving: 425 calories, 31 g protein,
59 g carbohydrates, 9 g fat SERVES 4
. . . .

Non-stick cooking spray

2 tsp extra virgin olive oil

2–3 cloves garlic, finely chopped

½ tsp chilli flakes

½ tsp dried Italian seasoning or oregano

½ tsp salt

¼ tsp ground black pepper

¼ tsp cayenne pepper

1 medium onion, chopped

450 g (1 lb) lean turkey mince

1 small green pepper, diced

230 g (8 oz) sliced mushrooms

750 g (1 lb 10 oz) pasta sauce from a jar

1 tin (400 g/ 14 oz) chopped tomatoes

4 tbsp Parmesan cheese

450 g (1 lb) wholewheat spaghetti or your favourite pasta

Note: *Omit the chilli flakes if you do not like it spicy.*

Heat the oil in a large saucepan; sauté the garlic, spices, salt and black pepper, cayenne pepper and onion for 2 minutes. Add the turkey and cook until browned. Next add the pepper and mushrooms; sauté for 4 more minutes. Add the pasta sauce and tomatoes and bring to the boil; reduce the heat. Simmer, uncovered, for 15 minutes, stirring occasionally. Stir the cheese into the sauce before serving.

Prepare the pasta according to the directions on the packet. For al dente pasta, take 3 minutes off the recommended cooking time.

Serve one quarter of the cooked pasta topped with red sauce per serving.

PROTEIN POWERED	CARBOHYDRATE CONCENTRATED	FAT FRIENDLY	FREE FOODS
Lean turkey mince	Wholewheat pasta	Extra virgin olive oil	Mushrooms, garlic, spices, onion, green pepper, tomatoes

Creamy Lemon Basil Chicken Linguine

Nutrition facts per serving: 386 calories, 31 g protein,
54 g carbohydrates, 5 g fat SERVES 4

• •

120 ml (4 fl oz) low-fat soured cream

120 ml (4 fl oz) full-fat milk

120 ml (4 fl oz) low-salt chicken stock

2 tbsp lemon juice

1½ tsp garlic, finely chopped

45 g (1½ oz) fresh basil

1 medium lemon, peeled and sliced (grate the peel)

¼ tsp crushed chillies

230 g (8 oz) wholewheat linguine

340 g (12 oz) boneless, skinless chicken breasts, cut into 1 cm (½ in) strips

Salt

Ground black pepper

Non-stick cooking spray

Basil leaves, for garnish

In a medium bowl, combine the soured cream, milk, chicken stock, lemon juice and garlic.

Chop the basil in a food processor.

Turn on the processor and slowly add the liquid mixture. Turn off the processor as soon as the bowl is empty.

Transfer to a saucepan. Stir in the lemon peel and crushed chillies, then set aside.

Cook the linguine according to instructions on the packet.

Season the chicken with salt and black pepper. Spray a frying pan with cooking spray, and heat on medium high. Brown the chicken on each side for 3 to 4 minutes, or until cooked through.

When the chicken and linguine are cooked, heat the sauce for 3 to 5 minutes over a medium–low heat. Do not allow to boil.

Toss together the sauce, linguine and chicken. Garnish with the lemon slices and basil leaves.

PROTEIN POWERED	CARBOHYDRATE CONCENTRATED	FAT FRIENDLY	FREE FOODS
Chicken breasts, milk	Wholewheat linguine	Cooking spray	Chicken stock, lemon juice, herbs, spices

Nutrition facts calculated by Menu Magic Personal Chef Software, Version 2.6, 2008, Kreotek, LLC, Rio Rancho, New Mexico.

Mediterranean Prawn Pasta

Nutrition facts per serving: 399 calories, 30 g protein,
48 g carbohydrates, 10 g fat SERVES 4

• •

230 g (8 oz) brown rice fusilli or spiral pasta
4 medium tomatoes, seeded and chopped
115 g (4 oz) spinach leaves
2 tbsp extra virgin olive oil
¼ tsp salt
¼ tsp ground black pepper
1 tbsp garlic, finely chopped
450 g (1 lb) raw prawns, peeled and deveined
1 tbsp lemon juice
4 tbsp chopped fresh basil
Peel of 1 lemon, grated

Cook the pasta according to instructions on the packet.

In a large frying pan over a medium–high heat, sauté the tomatoes and
spinach in the olive oil with the salt, pepper and garlic.

When the spinach has started to wilt, add the prawns, lemon juice and basil,
and cook until the prawns are pink.

Toss with the pasta and sprinkle with the lemon peel.

PROTEIN POWERED	CARBOHYDRATE CONCENTRATED	FAT FRIENDLY	FREE FOODS
Prawns	Brown rice pasta	Extra virgin olive oil	Tomatoes, spinach, garlic, lemon, basil

*Nutrition facts calculated by Menu Magic Personal Chef Software, Version 2.6, 2008,
Kreotek, LLC, Rio Rancho, New Mexico.*

CHRISTINE'S NUTRITION NUGGETS Prawns are a fantastic source of lean protein; however, if you have high cholesterol, you should avoid prawns and use clams or chicken breast. Prawns are a little high in cholesterol and only need to be avoided by people who have high cholesterol.

Christine's Born-Again Lasagne

Nutrition facts per serving: 467 calories, 34 g protein,
61 g carbohydrates, 8 g fat SERVES 12

Non-stick cooking spray

2 tsp extra virgin olive oil

2–3 cloves garlic, finely chopped

½ tsp crushed chillies

½ tsp dried Italian seasoning or oregano

¼ tsp ground black pepper

¼ tsp cayenne pepper

½ tsp salt

1 medium onion, chopped

450 g (1 lb) lean turkey mince

1 small green pepper, diced

230 g (8 oz) sliced mushrooms

750 g (1 lb 10 oz) pasta sauce

1 tin (400 g/14 oz) chopped tomatoes

425 g (15 oz) low-fat ricotta cheese

2 tbsp chopped fresh parsley + extra for garnish

2 egg whites, lightly beaten

9 dried wholewheat lasagne sheets (no pre-cooking required type)

450 g (1 lb) light mozzarella

60 g (2 oz) Parmesan cheese, grated

12 slices sourdough bread

Coat a large rectangular baking dish with cooking spray; set aside. Heat the oil in a large saucepan; sauté the garlic, spices, salt and onion for 2 minutes. Add the turkey and cook until browned. Next add the pepper and mushrooms; sauté for 4 more minutes. Add the pasta sauce and tomatoes and bring to the boil; reduce the heat. Simmer, uncovered, for 15 minutes, stirring occasionally.

Preheat the oven to 190ºC/375ºF/gas 5. In a medium bowl, combine the ricotta, parsley and egg until smooth, set aside. Cover the bottom of the prepared baking dish with 4½ of the lasagne sheets; then spread half of the ricotta mixture on top, followed by half of the meat sauce and a light layer of mozzarella cheese. Repeat the layering process.

Cover and bake for 40 minutes. Uncover. Sprinkle with the Parmesan and bake for 10 minutes. Let stand for 10 minutes before serving. Garnish with parsley.

PROTEIN POWERED	CARBOHYDRATE CONCENTRATED	FAT FRIENDLY	FREE FOODS
Lean turkey mince, ricotta	Wholewheat lasagne sheets, pasta sauce, tomatoes	Extra virgin olive oil, light mozzarella	Herbs, spices, onion, mushrooms, pepper

Wasabi Sesame Salmon with Brown Rice Noodles

Nutrition facts per serving: 400 calories, 25 g protein,
48 g carbohydrates, 12 g fat SERVES 4

SALMON

Non-stick cooking spray

425 g (15 oz) wild salmon,
cut into 4 pieces

Pinch of salt

Pinch of ground black pepper

60 g (2 oz) light mayonnaise

1 tbsp wasabi

1 tbsp black sesame seeds

NOODLES

230 g (8 oz) brown rice spaghetti

1 medium carrot, grated

4 tbsp low-salt soy sauce

4 tbsp low-salt chicken stock

½ tsp hot chilli sauce

3 spring onions, chopped

TO MAKE THE SALMON:

Preheat the oven to 190ºC/375ºF/gas 5. Spray a baking tray with cooking spray. Place the salmon on the pan and season with the salt and pepper.

Mix the mayonnaise and wasabi together and brush evenly on the salmon. Sprinkle with the sesame seeds. Bake for 7 to 10 minutes, or until the salmon is opaque.

TO MAKE THE NOODLES:

Cook the spaghetti according the directions on the package. One minute before draining, add the carrots.

Mix the soy sauce, stock and chilli sauce together. Stir the sauce into the drained noodles. Top with the spring onions.

PROTEIN POWERED	CARBOHYDRATE CONCENTRATED	FAT FRIENDLY	FREE FOODS
Salmon	Brown rice spaghetti, carrots	Light mayonnaise, sesame seeds	Wasabi, soy sauce, chicken stock, chilli sauce, spring onions

Nutrition facts calculated by Menu Magic Personal Chef Software, Version 2.6, 2008, Kreotek, LLC, Rio Rancho, New Mexico.

CHRISTINE'S NUTRITION NUGGETS Brown rice noodles offer an excellent alternative for people who suffer from coeliac disease, a wheat gluten allergy. They are also high in fibre, which is known to help stabilize blood sugar levels.

Sugar and Spice Salmon with Barbecue Sweet Potatoes

Nutrition facts per serving: 367 calories, 24 g protein, 51 g carbohydrates, 7 g fat SERVES 4

- -

SALMON

Non-stick cooking spray

2 tbsp brown sugar

2 tsp chilli powder

1 tsp cumin

1 tsp paprika

½ tsp salt

½ tsp ground black pepper

¼ tsp cayenne pepper

450 g (16 oz) wild salmon, cut in 4 pieces

SWEET POTATOES

60 ml (2 fl oz) barbecue sauce

60 ml (2 fl oz) low-salt chicken stock

4 medium sweet potatoes, cut into 5 mm (¼ in) rounds

Non-stick cooking spray

TO MAKE THE SALMON:

Preheat the oven to 190ºC/375ºF/gas 5. Spray a baking tray with cooking spray.

In a small bowl, mix all the dry ingredients together. Dust the top of each piece of salmon with the spice mix, then place in the prepared baking tray. Bake for 7 to 10 minutes, or until the salmon is opaque.

TO MAKE THE SWEET POTATOES:

Mix the barbecue sauce and stock together well. Gently stir the sweet potatoes in the sauce to coat well. Remove the sweet potato slices and place on a baking tray coated with cooking spray. Keep the potatoes in a single layer and use a second baking tray if needed. Bake for 15 minutes at 190ºC/375ºF/gas 5.

PROTEIN POWERED	CARBOHYDRATE CONCENTRATED	FAT FRIENDLY	FREE FOODS
Salmon	Barbecue sauce, sweet potatoes	Heart-healthy fat in the salmon; cooking spray	Spices, chicken stock

Nutrition facts calculated by Menu Magic Personal Chef Software, Version 2.6, 2008, Kreotek, LLC, Rio Rancho, New Mexico.

CHRISTINE'S NUTRITION NUGGETS Adding hot spices to your meals can help curb hunger, according to a study in the *British Journal of Nutrition*. Additionally, scientists at the State University of New York at Buffalo found that capsaicin (a compound found in chilli peppers) triggers your brain to release feel-good endorphins.

Citrus Plaice

Nutrition facts per serving: 385 calories, 27 g protein,
47 g carbohydrates, 10 g fat SERVES 4
. . . .

450 g (16 oz) plum tomatoes, diced
Juice and grated zest of 1 orange
50 g (1¾ oz) green olives, finely chopped
480 ml (16 fl oz) water
Salt, to taste
285 g (10 oz) quinoa, uncooked
2 tbsp extra virgin olive oil, divided
Non-stick cooking spray
450 g (16 oz) plaice (or cod, or other flaky white fish)
Ground black pepper to taste

Preheat the oven to 190ºC/375ºF/gas 5.

In a medium frying pan, combine the tomatoes, orange juice, orange zest,
olives and 1 tbsp of the oil. Cook for 4 minutes, then set aside.

In a medium saucepan, bring the water to the boil with a pinch of salt. Add
the quinoa and 1 tbsp of the oil; cover and cook for 2 minutes. Turn off the
heat; let it stand until the quinoa absorbs all of the liquid (about 5 minutes).

Spray a roasting tin with cooking spray, season the fish with salt and pepper,
and bake for 10 minutes.

Layer each plate with quinoa, then top with the fish and finally with the
tomato mixture.

PROTEIN POWERED	CARBOHYDRATE CONCENTRATED	FAT FRIENDLY	FREE FOODS
Plaice	Orange juice, quinoa	Green olives, extra virgin olive oil	Plum tomatoes, orange zest

 CHRISTINE'S NUTRITION NUGGETS Green olives and olive oil contain high amounts of compounds deemed to be anti-cancer agents, according to the *European Journal of Cancer Prevention*.

Coconut Curry Sea Bass over Red Lentils

Nutrition facts per serving: 344 calories, 25 g protein,
42 g carbohydrates, 9 g fat **SERVES 4**

Non-stick cooking spray

4 banana leaves or string
for tying up sea bass

1 leek

1 small red pepper

1 small yellow pepper

1 small orange pepper

¼ tsp ground cumin

15 g (½ oz) unsweetened dessicated
coconut flakes

340 g (12 oz) sea bass,
cut into 4 fillets

180 ml (6 fl oz) light coconut milk

1 tbsp agave nectar

450 g (1 lb) dried red lentils

Preheat the oven to 200ºC/400ºF/gas 6. Cover a medium-sized baking tray with foil and spray with cooking spray.

Cut off the edges of the banana leaves, if using, so that you have long strips of banana leaf to use as ties. If you do not have banana leaves, use string.

Slice the leek and peppers. In a shallow bowl, combine the cumin and dessicated coconut. Roll all sides of the fish in the coconut mixture to lightly coat.

Place one piece of fish, some of the leek slices and some pepper slices in a banana leaf. Put 1 tbsp of coconut milk and a drop of agave nectar on each piece of fish and roll up each fish fillet.

Tie two banana leaf strips or string around each fish fillet, place onto the prepared baking sheet and cook for 20 minutes.

While the fish is cooking, prepare the lentils according to the directions on the packet. While the lentils are cooking, place any extra vegetables, coconut milk and 1 tsp of agave nectar in a medium saucepan, and cook over medium heat for 5 minutes, stirring occasionally.

When the fish flakes easily, place each fillet on top of ¼ of the cooked lentils and top with the coconut curry veggie sauce.

PROTEIN POWERED	CARBOHYDRATE CONCENTRATED	FAT FRIENDLY	FREE FOODS
Sea bass	Red lentils	Light coconut milk, unsweetened dessicated coconut flakes	Banana leaves, cumin, peppers

Coriander Lime Sea Bass

Nutrition facts per serving: 338 calories, 25 g protein,
47 g carbohydrates, 5 g fat SERVES 4

4 fillets fresh sea bass (90 g/3 oz each)

Juice of 2 limes

½ bunch fresh coriander, chopped

Salt and ground black pepper to taste

2 tbsp extra virgin olive oil

480 ml (16 fl oz) water

¼ tsp turmeric

90 g (3 oz) raisins

1 tbsp chopped fresh ginger

180 g (6½ oz) dry (uncooked) couscous

Note: For a kick-start meal, swap the raisin couscous for brown rice.

Place the sea bass in a roasting pan and add the lime juice, coriander, salt and pepper. Cover with clingfilm and marinate for 1 hour in the refrigerator.

Preheat the oven to 180°C/350°F/gas 4. While the fish is marinating, prepare the couscous. Bring the oil, water, a pinch of salt, the turmeric, raisins and ginger to the boil; add the couscous. Cover and simmer for approximately 5 minutes or until the water is absorbed.

Uncover the sea bass and cook for 15 minutes or until the fish flakes easily.

Serve the sea bass over the couscous.

PROTEIN POWERED	CARBOHYDRATE CONCENTRATED	FAT FRIENDLY	FREE FOODS
Sea bass	Couscous, raisins	Extra virgin olive oil	Limes, coriander, turmeric, ginger

CHRISTINE'S NUTRITION NUGGETS Turmeric is a potent antioxidant with anti-inflammatory properties. Some evidence suggests that turmeric has the potential to act as an anti-cancer agent.

Cajun-Style Grilled Prawns

Nutrition facts per serving: 410 calories, 28 g protein,
50 g carbohydrates, 11 g fat SERVES 4

450 g (1 lb) peeled and deveined medium prawns

2 tbsp extra virgin olive oil

Juice of 2 lemons

4 tbsp Cajun spice mix

Salt and ground black pepper to taste

480 ml (16 fl oz) water

250 g (9 oz) uncooked brown rice

Non-stick cooking spray

1 lemon, cut into 4 pieces

In a shallow dish, marinate the prawns with the olive oil, lemon juice, Cajun spice mix and salt and pepper for 20 minutes at room temperature.

While the prawns are marinating, prepare the rice. Bring the water to the boil; add the rice, cover and simmer for approximately 17 to 20 minutes or until the water is absorbed.

Warm a frying pan over medium heat. Remove from the heat, spray with cooking spray and return to the heat. Add the prawns and cook for 2 minutes on each side, or until the prawns are pink.

Serve with the rice and garnish with the lemon.

PROTEIN POWERED	CARBOHYDRATE CONCENTRATED	FAT FRIENDLY	FREE FOODS
Prawns	Brown rice	Extra virgin olive oil	Lemon, Cajun spice mix, salt, pepper

CHRISTINE'S NUTRITION NUGGETS Prawns are high in vitamin D, which is important for increasing calcium absorption and thus increasing bone growth. Vitamin D has been shown to help prevent certain cancers, heart disease, diabetes and osteoarthritis.

Apricot Glazed Chicken with Spicy Quinoa

Nutrition facts per serving: 386 calories, 28 g protein,
47 g carbohydrates, 9 g fat SERVES 4

CHICKEN

Non-stick cooking spray

340 g (12 oz) boneless, skinless chicken breasts

80 ml (3 fl oz) low-salt chicken stock

75 g (2½ oz) sugar-free apricot spread

1½ tsp Dijon mustard

¾ tsp Worcestershire sauce

1½ tbsp low-cal French dressing

½ tsp garlic powder

QUINOA

285 g (10 oz) quinoa, uncooked

1 tbsp extra virgin olive oil

1–2 sticks celery, chopped

50 g (1¾ oz) chopped red pepper

45 g (1½ oz) chopped onion

1 tsp paprika

¼ tsp cayenne pepper

½ tsp salt

¼ tsp ground black pepper

TO MAKE THE CHICKEN:

Coat a frying pan with cooking spray and place over a medium–high heat. Add the chicken and cook until browned. Transfer to a baking dish and set aside.

Combine the next 6 ingredients in a medium saucepan over medium heat. When the ingredients are mixed well, lower the heat and simmer for approximately 5 minutes, or until the sauce is slightly thickened.

Spoon the sauce over the chicken and bake at 180ºC/350ºF/gas 4 for approximately 8 to 12 minutes, or until the chicken is cooked through.

TO MAKE THE QUINOA:

Cook the quinoa according to the instructions on the packet, adding the oil, celery, pepper and onion to the quinoa before cooking.

When the quinoa is cooked, stir in the paprika, cayenne pepper, salt and black pepper.

PROTEIN POWERED	CARBOHYDRATE CONCENTRATED	FAT FRIENDLY	FREE FOODS
Chicken	Quinoa, apricot spread	Extra virgin olive oil, cooking spray, French dressing	Chicken stock, Dijon mustard, Worcestershire sauce, spices, celery, red pepper, onion

Sicilian-Style Chicken and Rice

Nutrition facts per serving: 414 calories, 33 g protein,
56 g carbohydrates, 6 g fat SERVES 12

Non-stick cooking spray

2 tbsp extra virgin olive oil

2 cloves garlic, finely chopped

½ tsp oregano

¼ tsp cayenne pepper

¼ tsp salt

¼ tsp ground black pepper

1.4 kg (3 lb) boneless, skinless chicken breasts

145 g (5 oz) wholemeal flour

1 large onion, chopped

450 g (1 lb) large white mushrooms, sliced

3 medium green peppers, thinly sliced

700 ml (1¼ pints) water

1 tin (400 g/14 oz) chopped tomatoes

400 g (14 oz) brown rice, cooked

Coat the bottom of a 5.5-litre covered, heavy-based casserole dish with cooking spray. Place the olive oil on the bottom of the dish and add the garlic, oregano, cayenne pepper, salt and black pepper. Sauté for 1 to 2 minutes.

Wash and pat dry the chicken, then coat with the flour. Add one-quarter of the onion and the floured chicken to the casserole and cook until the meat is no longer pink. Add the mushrooms and peppers and the remaining onion and sauté for another 5 minutes.

Add the water and tomatoes. Stir several times to keep the ingredients from sticking to the bottom of the casserole. Cook on medium low for 1 hour and 15 minutes.

PROTEIN POWERED	CARBOHYDRATE CONCENTRATED	FAT FRIENDLY	FREE FOODS
Chicken breast	Brown rice, wholemeal flour, tomato sauce	Extra virgin olive oil	Mushrooms, peppers, onion, garlic, cayenne pepper

CHRISTINE'S NUTRITION NUGGETS Mushrooms are loaded with biotin, and this meal provides 6 microg of biotin per serving. Biotin in its physiologically active form attaches to enzymes that are required for the synthesis of fatty acids.

Mushroom and Artichoke Chicken Scaloppine

Nutrition facts per serving: 393 calories, 29 g protein, 48 g carbohydrates, 9 g fat SERVES 4

. . . .

CHICKEN SCALOPPINE

340 g (12 oz) boneless, skinless chicken, thinly sliced

½ tsp salt, divided

½ tsp ground black pepper, divided

2 tbsp extra virgin olive oil

120 ml (4 fl oz) dry white wine

225 g (8 oz) sliced mushrooms

90 g (3 oz) chopped shallots

1 tbsp omega-3 spread

1 tsp thyme

120 ml (4 fl oz) low-salt chicken stock

1 tbsp garlic, finely chopped

1 tin artichoke hearts in water, quartered

2 tbsp cornflour

2 tbsp water

1 tbsp chopped fresh parsley

WILD RICE

400 g (14 oz) cooked wild rice

Juice and grated zest of 1 medium lemon

TO MAKE THE CHICKEN:

Season the chicken with half of the salt and half of the pepper. Using the oil as needed, brown each side of the chicken in a large frying pan until cooked through. Remove the chicken and keep warm. Deglaze the pan with the wine, scraping the bottom until clean. Strain and set the liquid aside.

Meanwhile, in a frying pan, sauté the mushrooms and shallots in the omega-3 spread with the remaining salt and pepper, and the thyme. After 3 minutes, add the stock and garlic. Simmer for another 5 minutes, or until the mushrooms are soft. Add the artichokes and cook for 1 minute more. Stir in the liquid from the deglazed pan.

In a small bowl, mix the cornflour and water. Slowly add to the mushrooms while stirring. Cook until slightly thickened.

Stir the lemon juice and zest into the wild rice and serve with the chicken. Pour the sauce over the chicken and sprinkle with parsley.

PROTEIN POWERED	CARBOHYDRATE CONCENTRATED	FAT FRIENDLY	FREE FOODS
Chicken breast	Wild rice, artichoke hearts	Extra virgin olive oil, omega-3 spread	Herbs, mushrooms, shallots, chicken stock, cornflour, lemon

Nutrition facts calculated by Menu Magic Personal Chef Software, Version 2.6, 2008, Kreotek, LLC, Rio Rancho, New Mexico.

Chicken Kebabs on Lemon Grass Skewers with Rice

Nutrition facts per serving: 338 calories, 25 g protein,
47 g carbohydrates, 5 g fat SERVES 4

. . . .

450 g (1 lb) chicken breasts, cut into
8 pieces (use 2 pieces per kebab)

1 onion, cut into cubes

1 red pepper, cut into squares

4 tbsp teriyaki sauce

1 tbsp sesame oil

1 litre (1¼ pints) water

400 g (14 oz) jasmine rice

4 lemon grass sticks
(for use as skewers)

Olive oil cooking spray

2 lemons

In a large freezer bag, marinate the chicken, onion and pepper in the teriyaki sauce and sesame oil for 20 minutes at room temperature.

While the chicken marinates, prepare the rice. Bring the water to the boil; add the rice, cover and simmer for 20 minutes or until the water is absorbed.

Build your kebabs by alternating the chicken, onion and pepper on each lemon grass skewer. Spray the kebabs with olive oil cooking spray.

Grill until the chicken is cooked through, about 5 minutes on each side.

Garnish with half of a lemon on each plate.

PROTEIN POWERED	CARBOHYDRATE CONCENTRATED	FAT FRIENDLY	FREE FOODS
Chicken breast	Jasmine rice	Sesame oil, cooking spray	Lemon grass sticks, onion, red pepper, lemons

 CHRISTINE'S NUTRITION NUGGETS Lemon grass has been shown to reduce oxidative stress caused by free radical damage. Additionally, the aroma of lemon grass is known to have a calming effect on the central nervous system.

Grilled Chicken Fajitas with Mango Salsa

Nutrition facts per serving: 417 calories, 30 g protein, 56 g carbohydrates, 8 g fat SERVES 4

. . . .

4 tbsp lime juice

1 tsp chilli powder

1 tsp cumin

1 tsp garlic, finely chopped

1 tsp oregano

¼ tsp crushed chillies

400 g (14 oz) boneless, skinless chicken breasts, cut into 2-cm (¾-in) strips

2 sliced red peppers, cut into 1-cm (½-in) strips)

2 medium onions, sliced, cut into 1-cm (½-in) strips

230 g (8 oz) fresh salsa

½ medium mango, chopped

½ medium avocado, chopped

½ tsp salt

½ tsp ground black pepper

Non-stick cooking spray

8 corn tortillas

2 limes, sliced

60 g (2 oz) low-fat soured cream

Preheat a grill or barbecue. Whisk the first 6 ingredients together in a small bowl. Divide into 2 large freezer bags. Add the chicken to one bag and the peppers and onions to the other. Shake the bags to coat thoroughly. Leave to marinate for at least ½ hour.

In a medium bowl, combine the salsa, mango and avocado and set aside.

Season the chicken and vegetables with the salt and black pepper. Spray the grill with the cooking spray.

Grill the chicken until cooked through, approximately 4 minutes on each side. Grill the vegetables until brown, 10 to 15 minutes, turning frequently.

Wrap the tortillas in foil and place on the grill until warmed, 3 to 5 minutes.

Stuff the tortillas with the chicken, peppers and onion, and top with the mango salsa. Garnish with the lime slices and serve with the soured cream.

PROTEIN POWERED	CARBOHYDRATE CONCENTRATED	FAT FRIENDLY	FREE FOODS
Chicken breast	Corn tortillas, mango	Cooking spray, avocado	Lime juice, herbs, spices, peppers, onions, salsa, low-fat soured cream

Nutrition facts calculated by Menu Magic Personal Chef Software, Version 2.6, 2008, Kreotek, LLC, Rio Rancho, New Mexico.

Tex-Mex Chicken with Chipotle Sauce

Nutrition facts per serving: 345 calories, 23 g protein,
53 g carbohydrates, 9 g fat SERVES 6

TEX-MEX CHICKEN

450 g (1 lb) skinless, boneless chicken breasts, sliced

Juice of 2 limes

2 tbsp extra virgin olive oil

1 tsp chipotle adobo sauce or paste (from jar)

Non-stick cooking spray

1 mild onion, thinly sliced

1 yellow pepper, thinly sliced

1 red pepper, thinly sliced

PICO DE GALLO

230 g (8 oz) plum tomatoes, chopped

½ bunch fresh coriander, chopped

Salt and ground black pepper to taste

1 jalapeño chilli pepper, chopped, seeds removed

2 medium avocados

BLACK BEAN SUCCOTASH

685 g (1½ lb) frozen sweetcorn, cooked

450 g (1 lb) tinned organic black beans in water, drained

TO MAKE THE TEX-MEX CHICKEN:

Marinate the chicken breasts with the lime juice, oil and adobo sauce for a minimum of 1 hour in the refrigerator, covered with clingfilm.

Grill the chicken under a medium heat until cooked through, about 6 minutes on each side.

Coat a medium frying pan with cooking spray and sauté the onion and peppers for 5 minutes. Add the cooked chicken and set aside.

TO MAKE THE PICO DE GALLO:

In a bowl, combine the tomatoes, coriander, salt, black pepper and jalapeño pepper.

Peel the avocados and cut each into thin slices.

Arrange the chicken on six plates, cover with the pico de gallo and one-third of an avocado, and serve with a portion of sweetcorn and a portion of black beans. If you are not on the kick-start programme, you may also serve with 3 small corn tortillas per person.

PROTEIN POWERED	CARBOHYDRATE CONCENTRATED	FAT FRIENDLY	FREE FOODS
Chicken breast	Black beans, corn	Olive oil, avocado	Limes, chipotle adobo sauce, pepper, onion, plum tomatoes, coriander, jalapeño chilli pepper

Baked Turkey Chimichanga

Nutrition facts per serving: 392 calories, 27 g protein,
50 g carbohydrates, 9 g fat SERVES 2

• •

145 g (5 oz) lean turkey mince
1 pinch each of salt and ground black pepper
115 g (4 oz) fresh salsa
100 g (3½ oz) Mexican spicy refried black beans
2 tbsp green chilli peppers from a jar, diced
Non-stick cooking spray
2 large wholewheat tortillas
60 g (2 oz) low-fat soured cream

Preheat the oven to 190ºC/375ºF/gas 5.

Cook the turkey with the salt and pepper in a non-stick pan until almost done.

Add the salsa, beans, chilli and peppers and cook off any liquid from the salsa.

Spray a baking tray with cooking spray and lay the tortillas out flat.

Pour half of the turkey mixture into the middle of each tortilla, and roll up like a burrito.

Bake for approximately 10 minutes or until slightly crispy.

Serve with the soured cream.

PROTEIN POWERED	CARBOHYDRATE CONCENTRATED	FAT FRIENDLY	FREE FOODS
Lean turkey mince	Refried beans, wholewheat tortillas	Cooking spray	Salsa, green chilli peppers, low-fat soured cream

Nutrition facts calculated by Menu Magic Personal Chef Software, Version 2.6, 2008, Kreotek, LLC, Rio Rancho, New Mexico.

CHRISTINE'S NUTRITION NUGGETS Black beans are an excellent natural PC Combo food. Half a cup of refried black beans contains 6 grams of protein, 18 grams of carbohydrates, 7 grams of fibre, and 1.5 grams of fat. They are a fantastic food when it comes to keeping blood sugar levels stable.

Christine's Enchiladas

Nutrition facts per serving: 372 calories, 28 g protein, 54 g carbohydrates, 7 g fat SERVES 8

• •

1 tbsp extra virgin olive oil

2 cloves garlic, finely chopped

1 tsp crushed chillies

½ tsp cayenne pepper

1 tsp garlic salt

1 medium onion, diced

450 g (1 lb) extra-lean turkey mince

540 g (1 lb 3 oz) enchilada sauce

100 g (3½ oz) pitted black olives, sliced

4 tbsp chopped fresh coriander + additional for garnish

115 g (4 oz) diced green chilli peppers

230 g (8 oz) grated low-fat Cheddar cheese

16 corn tortillas (15 cm/6 in diameter)

400 g (14 oz) cooked brown rice

Salsa

Low-fat soured cream (optional)

Preheat the oven to 180ºC/350ºF/gas 4. Place the first 5 ingredients in an extra-large, deep frying pan and sauté for 1 to 2 minutes. Add one-quarter of the onion and all of the turkey. Cook until the turkey is completely browned.

Warm the enchilada sauce in a medium saucepan on low for 3 to 5 minutes. While the sauce is warming, in a large mixing bowl, combine the turkey mixture, the remaining onion, and the olives, coriander, chilli peppers and Cheddar. Set aside.

Coat a 32.5 x 23 cm (13 x 9 in) glass baking dish with cooking spray. Spread 170 g (6 oz) of the enchilada sauce over the bottom of the baking dish. Then, using a set of tongs, take one tortilla at a time and carefully cover both sides with the sauce. Place 75 g (2½ oz) of enchilada mixture into each wet tortilla and roll up. Place each enchilada seam-side down into the baking dish.

Once all 16 enchiladas are firmly placed into the baking dish, pour the remaining enchilada sauce over the whole dish of uncooked enchiladas. Cover with foil and bake for 20 minutes. Serve with 65 g (2¼ oz) steamed rice, salsa and low-fat soured cream (if desired), and garnish with extra coriander.

PROTEIN POWERED	CARBOHYDRATE CONCENTRATED	FAT FRIENDLY	FREE FOODS
Lean turkey mince, low-fat cheese	Rice, enchilada sauce, corn tortillas	Extra virgin olive oil, black olives	Coriander, onion, green chilli peppers, garlic, crushed chillies, spices, salsa, low-fat soured cream

Christine's Favourite Steak with Mushroom Sauce

Nutrition facts per serving: 360 calories, 27 g protein, 47 g carbohydrates, 5 g fat SERVES 4

BEEF

½ tsp each salt and ground black pepper

1 tsp chopped fresh thyme

½ tsp chopped fresh rosemary

4 cloves garlic, finely chopped

4 organic sirloin steaks (90 g/3 oz each)

Cooking spray

SAUCE

1 tsp extra virgin olive oil

½ tsp fresh thyme

230 g (8 oz) mushrooms (button or shiitake), sliced

4 cloves garlic, finely chopped

120 ml (4 fl oz) organic chicken stock

120 ml (4 fl oz) white wine

1 tbsp water

1 tsp cornflour

HERBY MASHED POTATOES

2½ large potatoes

150 ml (5 fl oz) organic chicken stock

1 tsp each freshly chopped thyme, chives and parsley

2 cloves garlic, finely chopped

2 tbsp low-fat soured cream

Salt and ground black pepper

Note: *If you don't have time to make mashed potatoes, you can substitute with 100 g (3½ oz) cooked brown rice per serving.*

TO MAKE THE BEEF:

Preheat the oven to 230ºC/450ºF/gas 8.

Combine the first 5 ingredients. Coat both sides of the steaks with cooking spray; rub steaks evenly with the thyme mixture. Place steaks in a roasting pan coated with cooking spray; cook for 8 minutes on each side, or until a thermometer inserted in the centre registers 63ºC/145ºF for medium-rare, 70ºC/160ºF for medium or 75ºC/165ºF for well-done. Remove from the oven; keep warm.

TO MAKE THE SAUCE:

While the steaks are cooking, heat the oil in a large non-stick frying pan over a medium heat. Add the thyme, mushrooms and garlic; cook for 5 minutes or until the mushrooms are tender. Add the stock and wine; bring to the boil. Cook until reduced by half (about 10 minutes).

Combine the water and cornflour in a small bowl, stirring with a whisk. Add the cornflour mixture to the pan; bring to the boil. Cook for 1 minute or until slightly thickened, stirring constantly. Divide the sauce among the four steaks.

TO MAKE THE POTATOES:

Peel the potatoes and cut them in half. Place them in a pan of cold water and cover. Bring to the boil over a high heat and simmer until the potatoes are tender when pricked with a fork, about 30 minutes. Drain.

Bring the chicken stock to the boil, then turn down to simmer. Mash the potatoes and combine with the stock, herbs, garlic and soured cream. Add salt and pepper to taste.

PROTEIN POWERED	CARBOHYDRATE CONCENTRATED	FAT FRIENDLY	FREE FOODS
Sirloin steak	Potatoes or brown rice	Extra virgin olive oil	Mushrooms, garlic, rosemary, thyme, cornflour, stock

California Fruit Kebabs

Nutrition facts per serving: 313 calories, 27 g protein,
46 g carbohydrates, 4 g fat SERVES 4
• •

8 cubes (2.5 cm/1 in each) watermelon
8 cubes (2.5 cm/1 in each) honeydew melon
8 cubes (2.5 cm/1 in each) cantaloupe
8 large strawberries, hulled
4 tbsp orange blossom honey
3 tbsp chopped fresh mint
4 lemon grass sticks to use as skewers
900 g (2 lb) 0% fat-free plain Greek yogurt
4 tbsp slivered almonds
4 whole mint leaves

In a large bowl, mix the fruit together and cover with the honey and chopped mint. Marinate for 20 minutes in the refrigerator.

Assemble the kebabs by alternating the fruit on the lemon grass sticks.

Grill under a medium heat for 2 minutes on each side.

Serve with the yogurt in individual bowls for dipping. Garnish the yogurt with the almonds and mint leaves.

PROTEIN POWERED	CARBOHYDRATE CONCENTRATED	FAT FRIENDLY	FREE FOODS
Greek yogurt	Watermelon, honeydew, cantaloupe, strawberries, honey	Slivered almonds	Mint

Low-Fat, Low-Sugar Pumpkin Bread

Nutrition facts per serving: 196 calories, 5 g protein,
44 g carbohydrates, 1 gram fat SERVES 8

Non-stick cooking spray

240 ml (8 fl oz) egg whites

250 g (9 oz) canned pumpkin

115 g (14 oz) unsweetened stewed apple

120 ml (4 fl oz) water

150 g (5½ oz) caster sugar

150 g (5½ oz) Splenda

245 g (8½ oz) wholemeal flour

1 tsp bicarbonate of soda

1 tsp ground cinnamon

¼ tsp ground cloves

¼ tsp ground nutmeg

¾ tsp salt

¼ tsp baking powder

1 tbsp chopped walnuts

Preheat the oven to 180ºC/350ºF/gas 4. Coat a 9x 5 in (900g/2 lb) loaf tin with cooking spray and set aside.

Combine the next 6 ingredients in a medium mixing bowl. In a large mixing bowl, combine the bicarbonate of soda, cinnamon, cloves, nutmeg, salt, flour and baking powder.

Pour the liquid mixture into the dry mixture and mix well. Pour into the prepared loaf tin and sprinkle the walnuts over the top. Bake for 40 minutes or until a toothpick inserted into the middle comes out clean.

Note: *You can also use three mini loaf tins instead of making one large loaf and give two of the loaves away as gifts. Just wrap them in coloured cellophane and tie with a festive ribbon.*

PROTEIN POWERED	CARBOHYDRATE CONCENTRATED	FAT FRIENDLY	FREE FOODS
Egg whites	Stewed apple, sugar, wholemeal flour	Cooking spray, walnuts	Bicarbonate of soda, cinnamon, cloves, nutmeg, salt, baking powder

CHRISTINE'S NUTRITION NUGGETS This pumpkin bread is a healthy alternative to the typical tea breads; however, it is not a PC Combo recipe. I often crumble it into my low-fat cottage cheese for a sweet mid-afternoon PC Combo meal. However you choose to eat it, make sure it is paired with a lean protein such as chicken breast, low-fat dairy or a low-carb protein bar.

Christine's Low-Fat, Low-Sugar Cheesecake

Nutrition facts per serving: 250 calories, 21 g protein, 27 g carbohydrates, 6 g fat SERVES 8

. . . .

CRUST

125 g (4½ oz) reduced-fat digestive biscuit crumbs

3 tbsp unsalted butter, melted

50 g (1¾ oz) Splenda

FILLING

900 g (2 lb) extra-light cream cheese, softened to room temperature

250 g (9 oz) Splenda

1½ tbsp fresh lime juice

¼ tsp salt

Whites of 6 large eggs

115 g (12 oz) fresh raspberries

Preheat the oven to 180ºC/350ºF/gas 4.

TO MAKE THE CRUST:

In a medium bowl, combine the digestive biscuits, melted butter and Splenda. Place the mixture into a 23 cm (9 in) or 15 cm (6 in) round cake tin and bake for 10 minutes.

TO MAKE THE FILLING:

In a large bowl, beat the cream cheese and Splenda until smooth using a hand-held electric mixer. Add the lime juice and salt; continue to beat until smooth. Add the egg whites one at a time, beating after each addition. Pour the filling over the base and bake for 50 to 60 minutes. Remember to turn the cheesecake halfway through the cooking process. Allow to cool and then refrigerate for 4 to 6 hours before serving. Top with the raspberries.

PROTEIN POWERED	CARBOHYDRATE CONCENTRATED	FAT FRIENDLY	FREE FOODS
Cream cheese, egg whites	Digestive biscuit crumbs, raspberries	Butter	Splenda

CHRISTINE'S NUTRITION NUGGETS This cheesecake is a PC Combo, but that doesn't mean you should eat it on its own. Enjoy this dessert with any dinner from the Skinny Chicks meal plans by reducing the proteins and carbohydrates to half the suggested portions. Since you get 27 grams of carbohydrates and 21 grams of protein from one slice of this cake, you need to eat only half of your recommended protein and carbs for your main meal.

Pineapple Carpaccio

Nutrition facts per serving: 217 calories, 2 g protein,
50 g carbohydrates, 2 g fat SERVES 4

. . . .

FRUIT
1 small fresh pineapple, peeled

SYRUP
90 g (3 oz) brown sugar

480 ml (16 fl oz) water

2 cinnamon sticks

1 rosemary stalk

Juice of 2 lemons

1 tsp rum extract

225 g (8 oz) low-fat vanilla ice cream

TO PREPARE THE FRUIT:
Slice the peeled pineapple into thin slices; arrange nicely on four large soup plates.

TO MAKE THE SYRUP:
In a medium saucepan, boil the brown sugar, water, cinnamon sticks, rosemary, lemon juice and rum extract for 5 minutes. Cover and allow to set until the syrup returns to room temperature.

Strain using a tea strainer.

Cover the pineapple with the syrup mixture and top with a scoop of vanilla ice cream.

PROTEIN POWERED	CARBOHYDRATE CONCENTRATED	FAT FRIENDLY	FREE FOODS
	Pineapple, brown sugar, low-fat vanilla ice cream (8 g carbs per serving)	Low-fat vanilla ice cream (2 g fat per serving)	Cinnamon sticks, rosemary sprig, lemon, rum extract

CHRISTINE'S NUTRITION NUGGETS This is a delicious dessert, but it should only be eaten with a low-carb meal because it contains 50 grams of carbs per serving. I enjoy a nice piece of grilled halibut and steamed vegetables for dinner and this pineapple carpaccio for dessert. A meal such as this makes for a delicious and fun PC Combo.

Raspberry Chambord Trifle

Nutrition facts per serving: 315 calories, 21 g protein,
49 g carbohydrates, 4 g fat SERVES 4

. . . .

450 g (1 lb) low-fat (2%) Total Greek yogurt
2 tbsp Chambord raspberry liqueur
6 tbsp brown sugar
450 g (1 lb) fresh raspberries
4 whole mint leaves

In a medium bowl, mix the yogurt together with the Chambord and the
brown sugar.

Layer in 4 clear, stemmed glasses, alternating yogurt, then raspberries, then
more yogurt and more raspberries.

Garnish with a mint leaf.

PROTEIN POWERED	CARBOHYDRATE CONCENTRATED	FAT FRIENDLY	FREE FOODS
Low-fat Greek yogurt	Liqueur, brown sugar, raspberries	Low-fat Greek yogurt	Mint leaves

CHRISTINE'S NUTRITION NUGGETS This dessert also works as a PC Combo. Feel free to omit the liqueur and serve to the whole family for a fun, delicious snack.

Sautéed Strawberries

Nutrition facts per serving: 213 calories, 1 gram protein,
52 g carbohydrates, 0 gram fat SERVES 4
• •

450 g (1 lb) seasonal strawberries from your favourite farmer's market
Non-stick cooking spray
2 tbsp demerara sugar
4 tbsp aged balsamic vinegar (preferably 20 years old)
480 ml (16 fl oz) fruit sorbet

Wash the strawberries; hull them and cut in half.

Spray a warm frying pan with cooking spray.

Add the strawberries and sugar and cook quickly over high heat, until the
mixture becomes slightly caramelized, approximately 2 minutes.

Add the vinegar and cook for 1 more minute on high heat.

Serve warm with a scoop of fruit sorbet.

PROTEIN POWERED	CARBOHYDRATE CONCENTRATED	FAT FRIENDLY	FREE FOODS
	Strawberries, sugar, sorbet		Balsamic vinegar

 CHRISTINE'S NUTRITION NUGGETS This dessert must be eaten with a low-carb meal, so just swap the carbs from any meal on the Skinny Chicks plan and enjoy.

Appendix

Food Lists

You can use these lists to create your own meals and for shopping purposes. Remember the portion guidelines:

Proteins: the size of your palm

Carbs: the size of your fist with the opposite hand wrapped around it, or a large fist

Fats: the size of a shot glass for nuts and half a shot glass for oils or creams

Kick-Start Plan Foods

PROTEIN

Beef

Organic, preferably grass-fed tenderloin or fillet steak

Poultry

Chicken breast

Turkey breast

Fish/Shellfish

All types, preferably wild caught

Sushi

Deli

Chicken

Turkey

Eggs

Eggs, whole (limit 1 per meal)

Egg whites, Two Chicks liquid egg whites

Cheese

Low-salt preferred

All flavours and types

String cheese, light

Yogurt/Dairy

Plain, fat-free or low-fat

Plain Greek, fat-free or low-fat, flavoured fat-free yogurt

Milk, skimmed

Soya milk, light

Vegetarian

Edamame

Lentils

Tofu, low-fat

Protein Powders and Bars

(Use sparingly.)

Egg white protein powder

Whey protein powder

Hemp protein powder

High-protein, high-fibre protein bar

CARBOHYDRATES

Fruits

All types and varieties, fresh or frozen

Pomegranate juice

Pumpkin, canned

Raisins, dried apricots, dates and prunes

Vegetables

All types and varieties, fresh, cooked, or frozen; this includes potatoes and yams

Legumes (pulses)

Black beans, lentils

Grains

Brown rice

Wild rice

Quinoa

Steel-cut (Scotch) oats

Sweetener

Agave nectar

Honey

Sauces

Enchilada sauce

FATS

Nuts/Seeds

All types, dry roasted or raw

Nut butters

Oils

Extra virgin olive oil

Canola (rapeseed) oil

Flaxseed (linseed) oil

Oil spray/cooking spray

Miscellaneous

Avocado

Black olives

Light mayonnaise

Unsweetened dessicated coconut

Coconut milk, light

Everyday Plan PC Combo Foods

PROTEIN

Beef
Organic, preferably grass-fed
Tenderloin or fillet steak

Poultry
Chicken breast
Turkey breast
Chicken or turkey, minced lean
Pork
Canadian bacon, fat-free or low-fat

Fish/Shellfish
All types, preferably wild caught
Sushi
Salmon burger

Deli
Chicken
Turkey

Eggs
Eggs, whole (limit 1 per meal)
Egg whites, Two Chick liquid egg whites

Cheese
Very low-fat only, except where indicated in recipe; low-sodium preferred
All flavours and types
String cheese, light

Yogurt/Dairy
Plain, fat-free or low-fat
Plain Greek, fat-free or low-fat
Milk, skimmed
Soya milk, light

Vegetarian
Edamame
Lentils
Seitan
Tempeh
Tofu, low-fat, firm or silken
Veggie burger, low-fat
Veggie slices, low-fat
Veggie hot dogs, low-fat
Veggie meat, minced, low-fat

Protein Powders and Bars
(Use sparingly) Chocolate, vanilla, strawberry or plain powder.
Egg white protein powder
Whey protein powder
Hemp protein powder
High-protein, high-fibre protein bar

CARBOHYDRATES

Fruits
All types and varieties, fresh, frozen or dried
Stewed apple, unsweetened
Pomegranate juice
Fresh homemade lemonade
Orange juice

Vegetables
All types and varieties, fresh, cooked or frozen
Tomato sauce, pasta sauce

Legumes
Black beans
Lentils

Grains
Brown rice
Couscous
Wild rice
Rice pilaf
Quinoa
Polenta

Breads
(Must be wholegrain or wholewheat)
Bread
Tortillas
Pitta
English muffin
Hamburger bun
Bagel

Cereal
Oats, steel-cut or rolled
High-protein cereal
Low-fat granola

Snacks
(Wholewheat or wholegrain)
Popcorn
Baked tortilla chips

Pasta
(Wholewheat or regular)
All pasta types, brown rice or regular

Tortillas
Preferably baked
Corn
Wholewheat

Yogurt
Flavoured, fat-free, all flavours

Sweetener
Agave nectar
Brown sugar
Maple syrup
Honey

FATS

Nuts/Seeds
All types, dry roasted or raw
Nut butters

Oils
Extra virgin olive oil
Canola (rapeseed) oil
Sesame oil
Oil spray/cooking spray

Miscellaneous
Avocado
Black olives
Omega-3 spread
Light mayonnaise

Skinny Chicks Free Foods

You can add these to any meal or eat these foods between meals.

VEGETABLES
LIMIT 1 SERVING RAW OR COOKED

Alfalfa sprouts
Asparagus
Aubergine
Bean sprouts
Broccoli
Cabbage
Cauliflower
Celery
Coleslaw (no dressing)
Courgette
Cucumber
Gherkin
Green beans
Kale
Kohlrabi
Leek
Lemons and limes
Lettuce, all types
Okra
Onion
Pak choi
Parsley
Peppers (jalapeño, red, green)
Pickles, dill
Radicchio
Radish
Sauerkraut
Spinach
Spring onion
Squash
Swede
Swiss chard
Tomato, raw
Tomato juice
Tomato sauce
Turnip tops
Turnips
Water chestnuts
Watercress

CONDIMENTS
LIMIT 1 TBSP PER SERVING

Balsamic vinegar
Barbecue sauce
Chicken stock
Cooking spray
Dressing, fat-free
Extracts
Hoisin sauce
Hot chilli sauce
Jams, low-sugar
Ketchup
Mustard (all types)
Parmesan cheese
Relish, gherkin
Rice vinegar
Salsa
Soured cream, low-fat
Soy sauce, low-salt
Spaghetti sauce
Tabasco
Wasabi
White wine vinegar
Worcestershire sauce

DRINKS

Coffee, plain, filtered water
Hot chocolate, sugar-free
Cola, diet
Tea, any flavour, unsweetened
Water, filtered or spring
Water, sparkling

HERBS AND SPICES
ALL HERBS AND SPICES CAN BE CONSIDERED FREE; THIS IS A LIST OF SKINNY CHICKS FAVOURITES

Bay leaves
Capers
Cayenne pepper
Celery seeds
Chilli powder
Chinese spice
Cinnamon
Cloves
Coriander
Crushed chillies
Curry powder
Garlic (all forms)
Ginger
Ground black pepper
Horseradish
Lemon pepper
Mint
Mustard seed
Nutmeg
Paprika
Rosemary
Saffron
Salt
Thyme
Turmeric
Vanilla
White pepper

References

CHAPTER 3

Whitney, Cataldo, Rolfes. 'Making Glucose from Protein.' *Understanding Normal and Clinical Nutrition,* 2002: 105.

CHAPTER 4

Ludwig, D.S., Majzoub, J.A., Al-Zahrani, A., Dallal, G.E., Blanco, I., and S.B. Roberts. 'High glycemic index foods, overeating, and obesity.' *Pediatrics.* 199; 103E26.

Pawlak, D.B., Kushner, J.A., and D.S. Ludwig. 'Effects of dietary glycaemic index on adiposity, glucose homeostasis, and plasma lipids in animals.' *Lancet.* 2004; 364: 778–85.

CHAPTER 5

Gold, P. et al. 'Decreases in rat extracellular hippocampal glucose concentration associated with cognitive demands during a spatial task.' *Proceedings of the National Academy of Sciences.* 2000; 97(6): 2881–85.

Jenkins, D. et al. 'Nibbling versus gorging: Metabolic advantage of increased meal frequency.' *New England Journal of Medicine.* 1989; 321: 929–34.

Kolata, Gina. 'Study Finds that Fat Cells Die and Are Replaced.' *The New York Times.* May 5, 2008. Retrieved online May 5, 2008 at http://www.nytimes.com/2008/05/05/health/research/05fat.html?scp-1&sq=Fat+Cell+Die&st=nyt.

CHAPTER 6

Groesz, L. et al. 'The effect of experimental presentation of thin media images on body satisfaction: A meta-analytic review.' *International Journal of Eating Disorders.* 2001; 31(1): 1–16.

CHAPTER 7

Due, A. 'Effect of normal-fat diets, either medium or high in protein, on body weight in overweight subjects: a randomized 1-year trial.' *International Journal of Obesity.* 2004; 18: 1283–90.

Feskanich D., Willett W.C., Stampfer M.J., Colditz G.A. 'Protein consumption and bone fractures in women.' *Am J Epidemiol* 1996; 143: 472–9.

Fittante, Ann, and the Editors of *Prevention* magazine. *The Sugar Solution.* New York: Rodale Inc., 2006.

Halton, T.L., Hu, F.B. 'The effects of high protein diets on thermogenesis, satiety and weight loss: a critical review.' *J Am Coll Nutr* 2004; 23: 373–85.

Sacks, F.M. et al. 'Soy Protein, Isoflavones, and Cardiovascular Health.' An American Heart Association Science Advisory for Professionals from the Nutrition Committee. *Circulation* 2006.

Vander Wal, J.S. et al. 'Short-term effect of eggs on satiety in overweight and obese subjects.' *Journal of the American College of Nutrition.* 2005; 24(6): 510–15.

Zemel, M. 'Regulation of adiposity and obesity risk by dietary calcium: Mechanisms and implications.' *Journal of the American College of Nutrition*. 2002; 21(2): 146S–151S.

Zemel, M. et al. 'Calcium and dairy acceleration of weight and fat loss during energy restriction in obese adults.' *Obesity Research*. 2004; 12: 582–90.

CHAPTER 8

Feskanich D., Willett W.C., Stampfer M.J., Colditz G.A. 'Protein consumption and bone fractures in women.' *Am J Epidemiol* 1996; 143: 472–9.

Gardner, C.D. et al. 'Comparison of the Atkins, Zone, Ornish, and LEARN diets for change in weight and related risk factors among overweight premenopausal women: the A TO Z Weight Loss Study: a randomized trial.' *Journal of the American Medical Association*. 2007; 297: 969–77.

'Hepatic Encephalopathy.' *The New York Times Health Guide*. Retrieved online May 28, 2008 at http://health.nytimes.com/health/guides/disease/hepatic-encephalopathy/overview.html.

Westman, E.C. et al. 'Effect of 6-month adherence to a very low carbohydrate diet program.' *The American Journal of Medicine*. 2002; 113(1): 30–36.

Whitney, Cataldo, Rolfes. 'Making Glucose from Protein.' *Understanding Normal and Clinical Nutrition*, 2002: 105.

CHAPTER 9

Albert, C. et al. 'Dietary α-linolenic acid intake and risk of sudden cardiac death and coronary heart disease.' *Circulation*. 2005; 112: 3232–38.

Bouchez, Colette. 'Want Healthy Skin? Feed It Well.' WebMD. Retrieved May 26, 2008 at http://www.webmd.com/skin-problems-and-treatments/features/want-healthy-skin-feed-well

Conklin, S. et al. 'Serum ω-3 fatty acids are associated with variation in mood, personality and behavior in hypercholesterolemic community volunteers.' *Psychiatry Research*. 2007; 152(1): 1–10.

Cromley, Janet. 'Eating Away at Illness.' *Los Angeles Times*. May 12, 2008. p. R3.

Gallagher, D. et al. 'Healthy percentage body fat ranges: an approach for developing guidelines based on body mass index.' *American Journal of Clinical Nutrition*. 2000; 72(3): 694–701.

Hill, A. et al. 'Combining fish-oil supplements with regular aerobic exercise improves body composition and cardiovascular disease risk factors.' *American Journal of Clinical Nutrition*. 2007; 85(5): 1267–74.

Mozaffarian, D., and E. Rimm. 'Fish intake, contaminants, and human health: Evaluating the risks and the benefits.' *Journal of the American Medical Association*. 2006; 296: 1885–99.

Whitney, et al. 'The Economics of Feasting,' *Understanding Normal and Clinical Nutrition*, 2002: 221–23.

CHAPTER 10

Brody, Jane. 'Personal Health: You Are Also What You Drink.' *The New York Times*. March 27, 2007. Retrieved online May 25, 2008 at http://www.nytimes.com/2007/03/27/health/27brody.html.

Cass, D. 'Kaiser Permanente Study Shows Alcohol Consumption—No Matter Beverage Type—Linked to Breast Cancer Risk.' Sept. 27, 2007. Retrieved online May 26, 2008 at http://ckp.kaiserpermanente.org/newsroom/national/archive/nat_070926_breastcancer.html.

Diepvens, K., Westerterp, K.R., and M.S. Westerterp-Plantega. (2006). 'Obesity and thermogenesis related to the consumption of caffeine, ephedrine, capsaicin, and green tea.' *Am J Physiol Regul Integr Comp Physiol,* July 13; [E-publication ahead of print].

Dulloo, A. et al. 'Efficiency of green tea extract, polyphenols and caffeine in increasing 24h energy expenditure and fat oxidation in humans.' *Am J Clin Nutri,* 1999; 70: 1040–5.

Goulding, Matt. 'The 20 Unhealthiest Drinks in America.' *Men's Health,* March 2008. Retrieved May 26, 2008 online at http://www.menshealth.com/eathis/Unhealthiest_Drinks_in_America/1_The_Worst_Drink_In_America.php.

Pearson, T. Alcohol and heart disease. *Circulation.* 1996; 94: 3023–35.

Whitney, Cataldo, Rolfes. 'Alcohol and Nutrition,' *Understanding Normal and Clinical Nutrition,* 2002: 231–33.

Whitney, Cataldo, Rolfes. 'Water Losses.' *Understanding Normal and Clinical Nutrition,* 2002: 388–89.

CHAPTER 12

Dietary Reference Intakes (DRIs), Food and Nutrition Board, Institute of Medicine, National Academy of Sciences 2004 (from website).

CHAPTER 13

Pelletier, C. et al. 'Associations between weight-loss-induced changes in plasma organochlorine concentrations, serum T3 concentration, and resting metabolic rate.' *Toxicological Sciences,* 67 (2002): 46–51.

Turpeinen, J.P. et al. 'Muscle fiber type I influences lipid oxidation during low-intensity exercise in moderately active middle-aged men.' *Scandinavian Journal of Medicine and Science in Sports.* 2006; 16(2): 134–40.

CHAPTER 15

Sohn, Emily. 'With Faux Sugars, Real Suspicion.' *Los Angeles Times.* Nov. 19, 2007. Retrieved online May 9, 2008 at http://articles.latimes.com/2007/11/19/features/he=sweet19.

APPENDIX

Goel, A. et al. 'Specific inhibition of cyclooxygenase-2 (COX-2) expression by dietary curcumin in HT-29 human colon cancer cells.' *Cancer Lett* 2001 172: 111–18

Kwon, Y.I. et al. 'Health benefits of traditional corn, beans, and pumpkin: *In vitro* studies for hyperglycemia and hypertension management.' *Journal of Medicinal Food.* 2007; 10(2): 266–75.

Acknowledgments

I owe my most special thanks to my husband and most special love, Neil Hazle, my ever-present sounding board, pseudo–writing partner (at many times) and best friend. You truly breathe life into me every day.

An endless thanks and love to all of my clients whose questions, answers, laughter, tears and completed food journals were the driving force behind this book. You have been my greatest teachers of all.

A huge thank you to my literary agents, Rusty Robertson and Sue Schwartz. Thanks for standing so firmly behind this book and going above and beyond at every juncture.

For the chance to finally place my life's passion into a book, a sincere thank you to Nancy Hancock.

An extraordinary, special thanks to Pam Krauss for your extra care and interest in my book and for being the most informative, professional and wonderful editor I could have ever hoped for. Because of you, this book sings.

To Sharyn Kolberg, your intent listening, understanding and articulation of my words has been a godsend. You truly blow me away. I'm blessed to have worked with you.

To all the chefs who contributed their amazing recipes to this book. A special thank-you to Chef Denise Macuk for bringing your awesome recipes to my clients and to this book, and to Chef Pierre Sauvaget, whose time and recipes have been invaluable.

My deepest gratitude to my friend and colleague William Smith of INTRAFITT, Inc. Your teaching, prayers, support, and positive energy helped set the blueprint for this book. William, your hard work and knowledge are truly altering the way Americans view weight loss – thank you for all that you do.

To Dr David Ludwig, for your important work in the area of obesity and for taking the time to discuss your studies with me.

To my dear friend Giuliana Rancic at *E! News*. Besides being an amazing client, you started the ball rolling and my life has never been the same. After all, you were the one who inspired me to expose those 'sinful salads'.

A very big thank you to everyone at Rodale: Beth Lamb, Beth Davey, Zach Greenwald and the entire group in New York and Pennsylvania for your help and support with the creation of this book.

To the Avanti Nutrition team: Jennifer Williams (junior nutritionist), Gaylie Felchlin (administrative assistant) and Hayley Morrisette (our hardworking intern), your can-do attitudes and teamwork are a blessing. Jen, thanks for being my right hand – you are the best!

To the gals who make me look so good. Melissa Brown is a miracle worker when it comes to beautiful hair – thank you for your amazing work and extreme professionalism. Vivanna Martin of Stila Cosmetics, you are truly heaven sent – thank you for fresh, clean makeup every time!

A loving thanks to my mom, my stepfather Chris, Janine, Lily Zukowski and Chris Green; you are my biggest heroes, supporters, listeners and fans. I can't imagine this life without your endless love.

To all my families who have always cheered me on: the Avantis, the Chiminellos, the Seatons, the Surfaces, the Hazles, the Busseys and the Bybees (especially you, Dad). A big hug to my wonderful aunts Mary, Louise, Gerry and Sandra. Thanks for your love, encouragement and never ending prayers. And of course, to my uncle John Chiminello, you are simply the best. Thanks for all your feedback via e-mail.

And most of all, I want to thank my wonderful Lord, Jesus Christ, who is always with me. Thank you for your favour and for taking me to new levels every day.

Index

Boldface page references indicate photographs. Underscored references indicate boxed text.

A

ABC&D concept, 18–20. *See also* Amount
    of food; Balance of blood sugar
    levels; Clock, eating around; Darnit,
    Get Your Lazy Butt on the Treadmill
Abdominal fat, 67, 113
Agave nectar, 215–16
Alcohol
    beer, 113
    body fat and, 112
    calories in, 113, 113, 115
    on empty stomach, 19
    in everyday plan guidelines, 137
    health benefits of, 113, 114
    health risks of, 114
    in kick-start plan guidelines, 120
    metabolism and, 112
    mixed drinks, 113, 113, 115, 115
    questions about in Skinny Chicks
        programme, 114
    red wine, 112–13
    weight loss and, 112
Amino acids, 42, 68, 125
Amount of food
    in ABC&D concept, 18
    calories and, 34–36
    dieting pitfalls and, 30–31, 34
    reasonable, 34
    semi-starvation theory and, 27–28,
        30
    starvation theory and, 24–27
Apples
    Apple Maple Pecan Parfait, 138
    Apple Raisin Oatmeal, 156
    Honey Nut Apple Crunch, 158
Apricots
    Apricot Glazed Chicken with Spicy
        Quinoa, 259
    Turkey Sandwich, Baby Carrots and
        Fruit, 138
    Veggie and Cheese Sandwich, 148
Artichokes
    health benefits of, 127, 163, 238
    Herb-Crusted Salmon with Baby
        Potatoes and Artichokes, 127
    Mushroom and Artichoke Chicken
        Scaloppine, 261
    Rosemary-Rubbed Salmon with Brown
        Rice and Steamed Artichoke, 163
Artificial sweeteners, 214–17
Asparagus

    Grilled Halibut with Quinoa and
        Asparagus, 159
    Grilled White Fish with Quinoa or Brown
        Rice and Asparagus, 129
Aspartame, 215
Avocados
    Cheese and Veggie Quesadilla, 142
    Grilled Chicken Coriander Lime Wrap,
        139
    Grilled Chicken Fajitas with Mango Salsa,
        145, 263
    Tex-Mex Chicken with Chipotle Sauce,
        135, 264
    Turkey Sandwich, Baby Carrots and Fruit,
        138
    vitamin E in, 153

B

Balance of blood sugar levels
    in ABC&D concept, 18–19
    carbohydrates and, 37–39
    FatEx analogy and, 39, 42
    nutrition and, 43
    PC Combo and, 37, 39
    protein/carb/fat formula and, 43–45
    satiety and, 43, 88
Bananas
    Chocolate Peanut Butter Smoothie, 162
    Hard-Boiled Eggs, Yogurt and Fruit,
        125
    Peanut Butter Toast, 144
Basil
    Bruschetta Chicken Wrap, 247
    Creamy Lemon Basil Chicken Linguine,
        250
    Mediterranean Prawn Pasta, 147, 261
B-complex vitamins, 166, 169
Beans and pulses, 75. *See also specific type*
    black, 276
    Chicken Soft Taco, 140
    Guiltless Turkey Nachos, 244
    pinto, 244
Beef
    Christine's Favourite Steak with
        Mushroom Sauce, 139, 267–68
    intake of, recommended, 69
Bingeing, 48–49, 84, 205
Biotin, 157, 270
Blood sugar levels. *See also* Balance of
    blood sugar levels

ABC&D concept and, 18–20
body image and, 57
erratic, 9, 12, 15
FatEx analogy and, 16–17, 30, 39, 42, 47
function of, 12–13
insulin and, 16–18
after meals, 47
in morning, 14
PC Combo and, 37, 39
stabilized, 17–18, 36
symptoms of fluctuations in, 9, 12
weight loss and, 9, 12
Blueberries
    Berry Delish Oatmeal, 146
    Blueberry Blinis, 238
    Blueberry Peach Smoothie, 130
    Blueberry Yogurt Parfait with Slivered
        Almonds, 150
    Fruity Bagel Dippers, 153
    Greek Yogurt with Honey and Walnuts,
        163
    health benefits of, 123, 130, 239
    High-Protein Cereal with Berries, 164
    Pomegranate Blueberry Greek Yogurt,
        122
    Wild Berry Parfait, 126
Body fat
    abdominal, 67, 113
    alcohol and, 112
    cells, 19, 50
    exercise in burning, 176–77
    visceral, 67
Body image
    blood sugar levels and, 57
    comparisons and, avoiding, 56, 58
    negative, 54–57
Body's fuel sources and tanks, 27, 28, 51,
    53
Bread
    Berry Good Stuffed French Toast, 241
    Blue Ribbon Cheese Burger, 144
    on empty stomach, 19
    Greek Chicken Pitta with Cucumber and
        Mint, 146
    Grilled Chicken Sandwich, 150
    Grilled Low-Fat Cheese Sandwich, 246
    healthy choices, 256
    Low-Fat Tuna Sandwich, 156
    Peanut Butter Toast, 144
    Sandwich and Baked Tortilla Chips, 154
    Sicilian Chicken Soup, 245
    Turkey Sandwich, Baby Carrots and
        Fruit, 138
Broccoli
    Baked Turkey, Sweet Potato and
        Steamed Broccoli, 161
    No-Fry Chicken Fried Rice, 248
    vitamin E in, 155
Brussels sprouts, 155

Butters, 100

C

Cabbage
    Asian Chicken Salad, 242
    No-Fry Chicken Fried Rice, 248
Caffeine, 108, 120, 137
Calcium, 73, 82
Calories
    in alcohol, 113, 113, 115
    amount of food and, 34–36
    in beer, 113
    counting, 34
    in juice, 107–8
    metabolism and, 18
    in mixed drinks, 113, 113, 115
    in salads, 8, 8–9
    sources of, 35–36, 43
Carb blockers, 174
Carbohydrates. See also PC Combo
    balance of blood sugar levels and,
        37–39
    building blocks of, 85
    complex, 85–86
    controversy of, 81
    daily intake percentage, 36
    diets low in, 14, 81–83
    eliminating, myth of, 37–39
    energy yields and, 37
    glucose and, 12–13
    glycaemic index and, 86–89, 87
    importance of, 85
    list of good, 287–88
    need for, 31
    PC Combo and, 89
    portion guidelines for, 44
    selections, healthy, 89
    simple, 85–86
    in Skinny Chicks programme, 89
Carrots
    Oven-Roasted Chicken Breast, Rice or
        Quinoa, Carrots and Courgettes,
        123
    Sicilian Chicken Soup, 245
    Thai Chicken Lettuce Cups, 243
    Turkey Sandwich, Baby Carrots and
        Fruit, 138
    Veggie and Cheese Sandwich, 148
    vitamin A in, 254
    Wasabi Sesame Salmon with Brown Rice
        Noodles, 143, 253
Celery
    Tuna-Stuffed Celery Sticks with Fruit,
        128
Cheese
    Blue Ribbon Cheese Burger, 144
    Cheese and Veggie Quesadilla, 142
    Christine's Born-Again Lasagne, 153,
        252

Christine's Enchiladas, 149, 266
Christine's Pasta and Spicy Red Sauce, 141, 249
Christine's Super Bowl Sunday Nachos, 158
Grilled Chicken Sandwich, 150
Grilled Low-fat Cheese Sandwich, 246
Guiltless Turkey Nachos, 253
healthy choices, 255
Onion and Tomato Egg White Scramble, 148
Sicilian Chicken Soup, 245
Spinach and Feta Scramble, 128
String Cheese and Fruit, 157
Super-Fast Tuscan Polenta, 160
Turkey and Cheese Roll-Up, 131
Veggie and Cheese Sandwich, 148
Cherries
Turkey Slice, Cherries and Trail Mix, 143
Chicken
Apricot Glazed Chicken with Spicy Quinoa, 259
Asian Chicken Salad, 242
BBQ Chicken Breast, Corn on the Cob and Melon, 130
Bruschetta Chicken Wrap, 247
Chicken Kebabs on Lemon Grass Skewers, 155, 262
Chicken Soft Taco, 140
Creamy Lemon Basil Chicken Linguine, 250
Greek Chicken Pitta with Cucumber and Mint, 146
Grilled Chicken Coriander Lime Wrap, 139
Grilled Chicken Fajitas with Mango Salsa, 145, 263
Grilled Chicken Sandwich, 150
Mushroom and Artichoke Chicken Scaloppine, 261
No-Fry Chicken Fried Rice, 248
Oven-Roasted Chicken Breast, Rice or Quinoa, Carrots and Courgettes, 123
as protein selection, popular, 69–70
Sicilian Chicken Soup, 245
Sicilian-Style Chicken and Rice, 165, 260
Tex-Mex Chicken with Chipotle Sauce, 135, 264
Thai Chicken Lettuce Cups, 243
Chilli peppers
Baked Turkey Chimichanga, 265
Christine's Enchiladas, 149, 266
Guiltless Turkey Nachos, 244
Tex-Mex Chicken with Chipotle Sauce, 135, 264
Chocolate
Chocolate Peanut Butter Smoothie, 162
dark, 212

Cholesterol, 49, 95, 100, 135, 261
CICO (Calories In Calories Out) theory, 24
Cinnamon
Apple Cinnamon Cottage Cheese, 141
Baked Yam Stuffed with Peanut Butter, Cottage Cheese and Cinnamon, 124
Cinnamon Raisin Oaty Muffins, 240
Pineapple Carpaccio, 272
Clock, eating around
in ABC&D concept, 19
blood sugar levels and, 47–48
body's fuel reserve tanks and, 51, 53
health benefits of, 49, 51
nighttime and, 53
principles behind, 48–49, 51
Skinny Chicks programme and, 46–47
Coconuts and coconut milk
Coconut Curry Sea Bass, 125
Coconut Curry Sea Bass over Red Lentils, 256
Thai Chicken Lettuce Cups, 243
Coffee, 108–9, 111
Cognitive improvement, 49, 99
Cooking food, 218, 228
Coriander
Asian Chicken Salad, 242
Christine's Enchiladas, 149, 266
Coriander Lime Sea Bass, 131, 151, 257
Grilled Chicken Coriander Lime Wrap, 139
Guiltless Turkey Nachos, 244
health benefits of, 151
Tex-Mex Chicken with Chipotle Sauce, 135, 264
Thai Chicken Lettuce Cups, 243
Corn
BBQ Chicken Breast, Corn on the Cob and Melon, 130
Cortisol, 67
Cortisol suppressants, 174
Cottage cheese
Apple Cinnamon Cottage Cheese, 141
Apple Maple Pecan Parfait, 138
Baked Nacho Chips and Cheesy Salsa, 152
Baked Yam Stuffed with Peanut Butter, Cottage Cheese and Cinnamon, 124
Blueberry Blinis, 238
Blueberry Yogurt Parfait with Slivered Almonds, 150
Cinnamon Raisin Oaty Muffins, 240
Fruity Bagel Dippers, 153
Peanut Butter Toast, 144
Pumpkin Pie Cottage Cheese, 129, 151
Wild Berry Parfait, 126
Courgettes

Baked Turkey Breast, Sweet Potato and
   Courgettes, 134
health benefits of, <u>250</u>
in Skinny Chicks programme, 123
Cream cheese
   Berry Good Stuffed French Toast, 241
   Blueberry Blinis, 238
   Breakfast Bagel Sandwich, 152, 160,
      239
   Christine's Low-Fat, Low-Sugar
      Cheesecake, 271
   Smoked Salmon Bagel, 157
Cucumbers
   Greek Chicken Pitta with Cucumber and
      Mint, 146
   as snacks, <u>139</u>
   Thai Chicken Lettuce Cups, 243
Cytokines, 98

D

Dairy products, 70, <u>73</u>, <u>145</u>. See also
      specific type
Darnit, Get Your Lazy Butt on the
      Treadmill, 19. See also Exercise
Deli meats
   Deli Slices and Fruit, 133, 161
   Turkey and Cheese Roll-Up, 131
Delis, eating at, 222–23
Dessert
   California Fruit Kebabs, 269
   Christine's Low-Fat, Low-Sugar
      Cheesecake, 271
   guidelines, 217
   Low-Fat, Low-Sugar Pumpkin Bread,
      270
   Pineapple Carpaccio, 272
   questions about in Skinny Chicks
      programme, <u>216</u>
   Raspberry Chambord Trifle, 273
   Sautéed Strawberries, 274
Detoxification, 121, <u>163</u>
DHA, 98–99, 172
Dietary fat
   'bad', 95–97
   daily intake percentage, 36
   diets low in, 91–92, 99
   energy yields and, 37
   essential fatty acids, 97–99
   in everyday plan guidelines, 136
   glycaemic index and, 39
   'good', 97
   importance of, 94–95
   in kick-start plan guidelines, 120
   list of good, 276–77
   monounsaturated, 97
   in nuts, 99–101, <u>101</u>
   omega-3 fatty acids
      defining, 97–99
      in fish, <u>72</u>, <u>143</u>

health benefits of, <u>143</u>
   supplements, 166, 169, 172–73
omega-6 fatty acids, 97–99
polyunsaturated, 97
portion guidelines for, 44
saturated, 95–96
'superhero', 97–99
trans fats, 96
triglycerides, 69
weight loss and, 92–94
Dieting
   Atkins diet, 37
   bingeing and, 84
   cabbage soup diet, 37
   drawbacks of, 14
   low- or no-carb diet, 14, 81–83
   low- or no-fat diet, 91–92, 99
   magazine articles about, 71, 73
   pitfalls, 30–31, 34
   starvation theory of, 18, 24–27
   Sugar Busters diet, 37
Diners, eating at, 223–24
Dining out
   casual restaurants/dining/takeout,
      223–24
   delis, 222–23
   fine dining, 224
   food stands, 222
   increase in, 218–19
   personal account of, 219, 222
Dinner
   Apricot Glazed Chicken with Spicy
      Quinoa, 259
   Baked Turkey, Sweet Potato and
      Steamed Broccoli, 161
   Baked Turkey Chimichanga, 265
   Cajun-Style Grilled Prawns, 133, 258
   Chicken Kebabs on Lemon Grass
      Skewers, 155, 262
   Christine's Born-Again Lasagne, 153,
      252
   Christine's Enchiladas, 149, 266
   Christine's Favourite Steak with
      Mushroom Sauce, 139, 267–68
   Christine's Pasta and Spicy Red Sauce,
      141, 249
   Citrus Plaice, 255
   Coconut Curry Sea Bass over Red Lentils,
      125, 256
   Coriander Lime Sea Bass, 131, 151,
      257
   Creamy Lemon Basil Chicken Linguini,
      250
   Grilled Chicken Fajitas with Mango
      Salsa, 145, 263
   Grilled Halibut with Quinoa and
      Asparagus, 159
   Grilled White Fish with Quinoa or Brown
      Rice and Asparagus, 129

Herb-Crusted Salmon with Baby
    Potatoes and Artichokes, 127
Mediterranean Prawn Pasta, 147, 251
Mushroom and Artichoke Chicken
    Scaloppine, 261
Oven-Roasted Chicken Breast, Rice or
    Quinoa, Carrots and Courgettes,
    123
Rosemary-Rubbed Salmon with
    Brown-Rice and Steamed
    Artichoke, 163
Sicilian-Style Chicken and Rice, 165,
    260
skipping, 27
Smoked Salmon Bagel, 157
Sugar and Spice Salmon with Barbecue
    Sweet Potatoes, 254
Tex-Mex Chicken with Chipotle Sauce,
    135, 264
Wasabi Sesame Salmon with Brown Rice
    Noodles, 143, 253
Docosahexaenoic acid (DHA), 98–99, 172
Dressings
    Christine's Asian Fusion Dressing, 242
Drinks, 105–7. See also specific type

E

Eating schedules, 225–26. See also Clock,
    eating around
EGCg, 173
Eggs
    biotin in, 157
    Hard-Boiled Eggs, Yogurt and Fruit, 125
    health benefits of, 248
    protein in, 70
    satiety and, 74
    yolks of, 70
Egg whites
    Berry Good Stuffed French Toast, 249
    Blueberry Blinis, 238
    Breakfast Bagel Sandwich, 152, 160,
        239
    Christine's Born-Again Lasagne, 153,
        252
    Christine's Low-Fat, Low-Sugar
        Cheesecake, 271
    Cinnamon Raisin Oaty Muffins, 240
    Egg White Salad in Lettuce Cups and
        Fruit Salad, 126
    Low-Fat, Low-Sugar Pumpkin Bread,
        270
    Low-Fat Egg White Salad and
        Crispbreads, 147
    Onion and Tomato Egg White Scramble,
        148
    with orange juice, 42
    protein in, 42, 243
    as protein selection, popular, 70

as side, 156
    Spinach and Feta Scramble, 128
    Veggie Delight Scramble, 132
Eicosapentaenoic acid (EPA), 98–99, 172
Electrolytes, 48
EPA, 98–99, 172
Ephedra, 173
Epigallocatechin gallate (EGCg), 173
Espresso, 109, 111
Everyday plan
    food lists, 288
    guidelines, 136–37
    meal plans, 14-day, 117–18, 138–65
    purpose of, 89, 136
Exercise. See also Workouts
    in ABC&D concept, 19
    beginner, 182–85
    body fat and, burning, 176–77
    heart rate and, 177–78, 180
    intermediate and advanced, 190–95
    muscle tone and, 180
    Skinny Chicks programme and, 175
    time of day for, 179
    water loss and, 107

F

Fat blockers, 174
Fat cell hypothesis, 50
Fibre, 129, 135
Fish and seafood
    Cajun-Style Grilled Prawns, 133, 258
    Citrus Plaice, 255
    Coconut Curry Sea Bass, 125
    Coconut Curry Sea Bass over Red Lentils,
        256
    Coriander Lime Sea Bass, 131, 151, 257
    Grilled Halibut with Quinoa and
        Asparagus, 159
    Grilled Salmon Steak with Rocket, 149
    Grilled Salmon or Turkey Steak on a Bed
        of Rocket with Lemon, 122
    Grilled White Fish with Quinoa or Brown
        Rice and Asparagus, 129
    Herb-Crusted Salmon with Baby
        Potatoes and Artichokes, 127
    Low-Fat Tuna Sandwich, 156
    Mediterranean Prawn Pasta, 147, 251
    mercury in, 70, 72, 133
    omega-3 fatty acids in, 72, 143
    as protein selection, popular, 70
    Rosemary-Rubbed Salmon with Brown
        Rice and Steamed Artichoke, 163
    Smoked Salmon Bagel, 157
    Sugar and Spice Salmon with Barbecue
        Sweet Potatoes, 254
    Sushi, Brown Rice and Steamed Veggies,
        132
    Tuna-Stuffed Celery Sticks with Fruit,
        128

Wasabi Sesame Salmon with Brown Rice
Noodles, 143, 253
Fish oil, 98, _161_
Fit and Lean Vegetarian programme, 75
Fizzy drinks, 229–30
Flaxseed (linseed), _129_
Food labels, 44, 167
Food lists, 43, 78–79, 276–78
Food logs, _76–77_, 84, 92–93
Food packaging, 213
Food stands, eating at, 222
'Free' foods, 121, 137, 278
Frozen meals, 162
Fruits, 119–21, _130_, 137. *See also specific
type*

G

Garlic, _147_, _257_
Ghrelin, 18, 26–27
GI, 39, 86–89, _87_
Ginger
Christine's High-Protein Pumpkin Ginger
Pancakes, 237
Coriander Lime Sea Bass, 131, 151, 257
health benefits of, _258_
No-Fry Chicken Fried Rice, 248
Glucagon, 69
Glucose, 12–13, 15–16, 19, 26, 42, 47, 51,
82, 86
Glycaemic index (GI), 39, 86–89, _87_
Glycogenolysis, 51
Grapes
Greek Chicken Pitta with Cucumber and
Mint, 146
in Skinny Chicks programme, 123
String Cheese and Fruit, 157
Green tea, 109
Green tea extract, 173

H

Hair health, 25, 68, 99
Heart health, 98, _100_, _114_
Heart rate, 177–78, 180
Honey
Greek Yogurt with Honey and Walnuts,
163
Honey Nut Apple Crunch, 158
Honeydew melon
California Fruit Kebabs, 135, 269
Hoodia, 174
Hormones, 26
Hunger, 21, 23, _104_
Hyperglycaemia, 16
Hypoglycaemia, 27, _29_, 30–31

I

Ice cream
Pineapple Carpaccio, 272
Insulin, 16–18, 30, 42, 69, 86–87

J

Joint health, 98
Juice, 38, 42, 107–8

K

Ketosis, 25, 82, _83_
Kick-start plan
benefits of, 119
food lists, 276
guidelines, 119–21
meal plans, 7-day, 117–18, _122–35_
purpose of, 89, 119
Krebs Cycle, 176

L

LDL cholesterol, 95, _100_
Lemon grass
California Fruit Kebabs, 269
Chicken Kebabs on Lemon Grass
Skewers, 155, 262
health benefits of, _273_
Lemons and lemon juice
Cajun-Style Grilled Prawns, 133, 258
Creamy Lemon Basil Chicken Linguine,
250
Grilled Salmon or Turkey Steak on a Bed
of Rocket with Lemon, 122
Pineapple Carpaccio, 272
Lentils
Coconut Curry Sea Bass, 125
Coconut Curry Sea Bass over Red Lentils,
256
Lettuce
Asian Chicken Salad, 242
Egg White Salad in Lettuce Cups and
Fruit Salad, 126
Thai Chicken Lettuce Cups, 243
Limes and lime juice
Christine's Low-Fat, Low-Sugar
Cheesecake, 271
Coriander Lime Sea Bass, 131, 151, 257
Grilled Chicken Coriander Lime Wrap,
139
Grilled Chicken Fajitas with Mango
Salsa, 145, 263
Tex-Mex Chicken with Chipotle Sauce,
135, 264
Lipase, 69
Lipoprotein lipase, 17

M

Macronutrients, 37. *See also*
Carbohydrates; Dietary Fat; Protein
Mango
Egg White Salad in Lettuce Cups and
Fruit Salad, 126
Grilled Chicken Coriander Lime Wrap,
139

Grilled Chicken Fajitas with Mango
  Salsa, 145, 263
Maple syrup
  Apple Maple Pecan Parfait, 138
  Christine's High-Protein Pumpkin Ginger
    Pancakes, 237
Marketing of food, 213
Meal plans. *See also specific meal*
  advantage of, 45
  everyday plan's 14-day, 117–18, 138–65
  kick-start plan's 7-day, 117–18, 122–35
  nutrition listings, 120
Meals, skipping, 15, 18, 24, 27
Meats, 68. *See also specific type*
Melon
  BBQ Chicken Breast, Corn on the Cob
    and Melon, 130
  California Fruit Kebabs, 135, 269
Mercury in fish, 70, 72, 133
Metabolism
  alcohol and, 112
  body fat cells and, 19
  calories and, 18
  defining, 28
  fast, 28
  muscle cells and, 19
  protein and, 67
  rate of, 18, 51, 53
  slow, 27–28
  starvation and, 19, 25
Milk
  Berry Delish Oatmeal, 146
  Christine's High-Protein Pumpkin Ginger
    Pancakes, 237
  Creamy Lemon Basil Chicken Linguine,
    250
  High-Protein Cereal with Berries, 164
Minerals, 167–68. *See also specific type*
Mint
  Berry Good Stuffed French Toast, 241
  California Fruit Kebabs, 135, 269
  Greek Chicken Pitta with Cucumber and
    Mint, 146
  Raspberry Chambord Trifle, 273
Mood boost, 98–99
Multivitamins, 166, 168–69
Muscles, 19, 25, 176–77, 180
Mushrooms
  Christine's Born-Again Lasagne, 153,
    252
  Christine's Favourite Steak with
    Mushroom Sauce, 139, 267–68
  Christine's Pasta and Spicy Red Sauce,
    141, 249
  health benefits of, 270
  Mushroom and Artichoke Chicken
    Scaloppine, 261
  Sicilian-Style Chicken and Rice, 165,
    260

Veggie Delight Scramble, 132

N

Nectarines
  Deli Slices and Fruit, 133, 161
  High-Fibre, Low-Fat Protein Bar and
    Fruit, 123
Negative thinking, 54–57
Nutrition
  balance of blood sugar levels and, 43
  challenge of, 14
  defining, 42–43
  effects of lack of, 25, 26
  health and, 45
  for meal plans, 120
  PC Combo and, 45
  Skinny Chicks programme and, 37
Nuts
  Apple Maple Pecan Parfait, 138
  Blueberry Yogurt Parfait with Slivered
    Almonds, 150
  California Fruit Kebabs, 269
  dietary fat in, 99–101, 101
  Greek Yogurt with Honey and Walnuts,
    163
  Honey Nut Apple Crunch, 158
  Low-Fat, Low-Sugar Pumpkin Bread,
    270
  protein in, 100–101, 101
  satiety and, 101

O

Oat flour, 246
Oats
  Apple Raisin Oatmeal, 156
  Berry Delish Oatmeal, 146
  Cinnamon Raisin Oaty Muffins, 240
  fibre in, 135
  Steel-Cut (Scotch) Oats with Side of
    Sweet Yogurt, 134
Obesity epidemic, 31, 109
Oils, 120, 161
Olive oil, 161
Olives
  Baked Nacho Chips and Cheesy Salsa,
    152
  Christine's Enchiladas, 149, 266
  Citrus Plaice, 255
  health benefits of, 255
Oranges
  Citrus Plaice, 255
  Citrus-y Greek Yogurt, 127
  juice, 38, 42
  Thai Chicken Lettuce Cups, 243
Overeating, 30

P

Pasta
  brown rice noodles, 253

Christine's Born-Again Lasagne, 153, 252
Christine's Pasta and Spicy Red Sauce, 141, 249
Creamy Lemon Basil Chicken Linguine, 250
image of, 65–66
Mediterranean Prawn Pasta, 147, 251
Sicilian Chicken Soup, 245
Wasabi Sesame Salmon with Brown Rice Noodles, 143, 253
PC Combo
blood sugar levels and, 37, 39
carbohydrates and, 89
Christine's Low-Fat, Low-Sugar Cheesecake and, 271
in everyday plan guidelines, 136
food list, 288
in kick-start plan guidelines, 119
nutrition and, 45
Pineapple Carpaccio and, 272
protein and, 67
Raspberry Chambord Trifle and, 273
Skinny Chicks programme and, 67, 89
in vegetarian diet, 74
weight loss and, 68
Peaches
Blueberry Peach Smoothie, 130
Deli Slices and Fruit, 133, 161
Tuna-Stuffed Celery Sticks with Fruit, 128
Peanut butter
Baked Yam Stuffed with Peanut Butter, Cottage Cheese and Cinnamon, 124
Chocolate Peanut Butter Smoothie, 162
Peanut Butter Toast, 144
Thai Chicken Lettuce Cups, 243
Pears
High-Fibre, Low-Fat Protein Bar with Anjou Pear, 155
Peppers
Asian Chicken Salad, 242
Chicken Kebabs on Lemon Grass Skewers, 155, 262
Christine's Born-Again Lasagne, 153, 252
Christine's Pasta and Spicy Red Sauce, 141, 249
Coconut Curry Sea Bass over Red Lentils, 256
Grilled Chicken Fajitas with Mango Salsa, 145, 263
No-Fry Chicken Fried Rice, 248
Sicilian-Style Chicken and Rice, 165, 260
Tex-Mex Chicken with Chipotle Sauce, 135, 264

vitamin C in, 155
Pineapples
Egg White Salad in Lettuce Cups and Fruit Salad, 126
Pineapple Carpaccio, 272
Pizza, 159
Polenta
Super-Fast Tuscan Polenta, 160
Pomegranates and pomegranate juice
health benefits of, 123
Pomegranate Blueberry Greek Yogurt, 122
Popcorn, 165
Pork, 69
Portion guidelines, 44, 136, 275
Portion sizes, 31
Potatoes
baked, 87
Baked Turkey, Sweet Potato and Steamed Broccoli, 161
Baked Turkey Breast, Sweet Potato and Courgettes, 134
Baked Yam Stuffed with Peanut Butter, Cottage Cheese and Cinnamon, 124
Christine's Favourite Steak with Mushroom Sauce, 267–68
Herb-Crusted Salmon with Baby Potatoes and Artichokes, 127
Herby Potatoes, 139, 267–68
Spinach and Feta Scramble, 128
Sugar and Spice Salmon with Barbecue Sweet Potatoes, 254
Veggie Delight Scramble, 132
Prawns, 261, 268. See also Fish and seafood
Pretzels, 213
Protein. See also PC Combo
belly fat and, 67
cortisol and, 67
daily intake percentage, 36, 43
in eggs, 70
in egg whites, 42, 243
energy yields and, 37
in everyday plan guidelines, 136
excess of, 82
fat burning and, 68–69
glycaemic index and, 39
health benefits of, 68
importance of, 66, 74
in kick-start plan guidelines, 119–20
list of good, 78–79, 287–88
magazine article diets and, 71, 73–74
metabolism and, 66
in nuts, 100–101, 101
PC Combo and, 67
portion guidelines for, 44
in prawns, 261
satiety and, 125

selections, popular, 69–70, <u>71</u>
in vegetarian diet, 74–75, <u>76–77</u>, 78
weight loss and, 68–69
Protein bar
High-Fibre, Low-Fat Protein Bar and Fruit, 123
High-Fibre, Low-Fat Protein Bar with Anjou Pear, 155
Protein/carb/fats formula, 43–45, 85
Protein powder
Berry Delish Oatmeal, 146
Blueberry Peach Smoothie, 130
Chocolate Peanut Butter Smoothie, 162
Christine's High-Protein Pumpkin Ginger Pancakes, 237
Cinnamon Raisin Oaty Muffins, 240
Pumpkin
Christine's High-Protein Pumpkin Ginger Pancakes, 237
health benefits of, <u>151</u>
Low-Fat, Low-Sugar Pumpkin Bread, 270
Pumpkin Pie Cottage Cheese, 129, 151

Q
Quinoa
Apricot Glazed Chicken with Spicy Quinoa, 259
Citrus Plaice, 255
Grilled Halibut with Quinoa and Asparagus, 159
Grilled White Fish with Quinoa or Brown Rice and Asparagus, 129
health benefits of, <u>159</u>
Oven-Roasted Chicken Breast, Rice or Quinoa, Carrots and Courgettes, 123

R
Raisins
Apple Raisin Oatmeal, 156
Cinnamon Raisin Oaty Muffins, 240
Raspberries
Berry Good Stuffed French Toast, 241
Christine's Low-Fat, Low-Sugar Cheesecake, 271
Grilled White Fish with Quinoa or Brown Rice and Asparagus, 129
Restaurants, eating at casual and fine dining, 223–24
Rice
Asian Chicken Salad, 242
Cajun-Style Grilled Prawns, 133, 258
Chicken Kebabs on Lemon Grass

Skewers, 155, 262
Christine's Enchiladas, 149, 266
Grilled White Fish with Quinoa or Brown Rice and Asparagus, 129
No-Fry Chicken Fried Rice, 248
Oven-Roasted Chicken Breast, Rice or Quinoa, Carrots and Courgettes, 123
Rosemary-Rubbed Salmon with Brown Rice and Steamed Artichoke, 163
Sicilian-Style Chicken and Rice, 165, 260
Sushi, Brown Rice and Steamed Veggies, 132
Thai Chicken Lettuce Cups, 243
white, <u>87</u>
Rocket
Grilled Salmon Steak with Rocket, 149
Grilled Salmon or Turkey Steak on a Bed of Rocket with Lemon, 122
vitamin A in, <u>149</u>
Rosemary
Pineapple Carpaccio, 272
Rosemary-Rubbed Salmon with Brown Rice and Steamed Artichoke, 163

S
Salads
Asian Chicken Salad, 242
calories in, 8, <u>8–9</u>
Cobb, 8, <u>8</u>
healthy, <u>242</u>
mentality about, 3–5, 7
weight loss and, 7–9
Salmon, <u>143</u>. *See also* Fish and seafood
Salsa
Baked Nacho Chips and Cheesy Salsa, 152
Baked Turkey Chimichanga, 265
Grilled Chicken Fajitas with Mango Salsa, 145, 263
Salt, 48
Satiety, 43, <u>74</u>, 88, 101, <u>125</u>
Sedentary lifestyle, 31
Semi-starvation theory, 27–28, 30
Serotonin, 99
Shopping for food, 228
Skin health, 25, 68, 99, 120
Skinny Chicks programme. *See also* Everyday plan; Kick-start plan
ABC&D concept of blood sugar levels and, 18–20
bingeing and, 205
body's fuel sources and, 27, <u>28</u>
carbohydrates in, 89
Clock and, eating around, 46–47
exercise and, 117, 175
goal of, 14
hunger and, elimination of, 21, 23, <u>104</u>
nutrition and, 37

overview of, 13
PC Combo and, 67, 89
personal accounts of transformation
  Casey F., <u>201</u>
  Courtney H., <u>208</u>
  Dianne M., <u>32–33</u>, **33**
  Dr John, 229–30
  Jeanne M., <u>90</u>
  Jennifer H., <u>102–3</u>, **103**
  Jennifer K., <u>220–21</u>
  Jessica C., <u>10–11</u>, **11**
  Joleen, 92–94
  Joy L., <u>110–11</u>, **111**
  Julia S., <u>6</u>
  Kallissa, 226–27
  Kate B., <u>80</u>
  Lezlie W., <u>40–41</u>, **41**
  Melida N., <u>58–59</u>, **49**
  Michelle E., <u>170–71</u>, **171**
  Nichole H., 75, <u>76–77</u>, 78
  Rachelle, 219, 222
  Raha T., <u>52</u>
  Rancic, Giuliana, 20–21
  Ruth W., <u>22</u>
principles behind, 19–20, 67
Q&A
  alcohol, <u>114</u>
  counting calories, <u>34</u>
  dessert, <u>216</u>
  fat cells, 50
  hunger, <u>104</u>
  hypoglycaemia, <u>29</u>
  mercury in fish and seafood, <u>72</u>
  time of day for exercise, <u>179</u>
  weight loss, <u>56</u>
in real life, 205–9
results of following, 57
'skinny' definition and, 13
sweets and, 211–13
as way of life, 210
weight loss and, 117, 207
Sleep, 53
Snap peas
  Asian Chicken Salad, 242
Social engagements and eating, 226–28
Sodium, 48
Sorbet
  Sautéed Strawberries, 274
Soured cream
  Baked Turkey Chimichanga, 265
  Creamy Lemon Basil Chicken Linguine, 250
  Grilled Chicken Fajitas with Mango Salsa, 145, 263
Spices, <u>254</u>
Spinach
  Bruschetta Chicken Wrap, 247
  Mediterranean Prawn Pasta, 147, 251
  Spinach and Feta Scramble, 128

Veggie Delight Scramble, 132
Splenda
  Christine's Low-Fat, Low-Sugar Cheesecake, 271
  Low-Fat, Low-Sugar Pumpkin Bread, 270
Spring onions, <u>245</u>
Starvation theory, 18, 24–27, 47, 49
Strawberries
  Berry Delish Oatmeal, 146
  California Fruit Kebabs, 135, 269
  Low-Fat Egg White Salad and Crispbreads, 147
  Sautéed Strawberries, 274
  Steel-Cut (Scotch) Oats with Side of Sweet Yogurt, 134
  Wild Berry Parfait, 126
Sucralose, 215
Sugar
  artificial sweeteners, 214–17
  cravings, 3–5, 7
  in juice, 107
  Low-Fat, Low-Sugar Pumpkin Bread, 270
  Pineapple Carpaccio, 272
  Raspberry Chambord Trifle, 273
  Sautéed Strawberries, 274
  Sugar and Spice Salmon with Barbecue Sweet Potatoes, 254
Supplements. *See also specific type*
  B-complex, 166, 169
  detoxification and, 121
  in everyday plan guidelines, 137
  fish oil, 98
  in kick-start plan guidelines, 121
  multivitamin, 166, 168–69
  omega-3 fatty acid, 166, 169, 172–73
  required, list of, 168
  vitamin deficiencies and, 167
  weight-loss, 173–74
Sushi, <u>133</u>, 164. *See also* Fish and seafood
Sweets, 211–13. *See also* Dessert

T

Takeaway food, 223–24
Target heart rate (THR) zone, 177–78
Tea, 109, 120, <u>139</u>
Thermogenic fat burners, 173–74
THR zone, 177–78
Thyroid increasers, 174
Tomatoes
  Breakfast Bagel Sandwich, 152, 160, 239
  Bruschetta Chicken Wrap, 247
  Christine's Born-Again Lasagne, 153, 252
  Christine's Pasta and Spicy Red Sauce, 141, 249
  Citrus Plaice, 255

Grilled Low-fat Cheese Sandwich, 246
Guiltless Turkey Nachos, 244
health benefits of, 141, 239
Mediterranean Prawn Pasta, 147, 251
Onion and Tomato Egg White Scramble, 148
Tex-Mex Chicken with Chipotle Sauce, 264
Topical weight-loss creams, gels and sprays, 174
Toxins, removing, 120, 163
Trail mix
  Turkey Slice, Cherries and Trail Mix, 143
Turkey
  Baked Turkey, Sweet Potato and Steamed Broccoli, 161
  Baked Turkey Breast, Sweet Potato and Courgettes, 134
  Baked Turkey Chimichanga, 265
  Blue Ribbon Cheese Burger, 144
  Breakfast Bagel Sandwich, 152, 160, 239
  Christine's Born-Again Lasagne, 153, 252
  Christine's Enchiladas, 149, 266
  Christine's Pasta and Spicy Red Sauce, 141, 249
  Grilled Salmon or Turkey Steak on a Bed of Rocket with Lemon, 122
  Guiltless Turkey Nachos, 244
  as protein selection, popular, 69–70
  Sandwich and Baked Tortilla Chips, 154
  Turkey and Cheese Roll-Up, 131
  Turkey Slice, Cherries and Trail Mix, 143
  Turkey Sandwich, Baby Carrots and Fruit, 138
Turmeric, 267

V

Vegetables, 119–21, 137, 258. See also specific type
Vegetarian diet, 74–75, 76–77, 78
Vitamin A, 149, 254, 280
Vitamin C, 155, 239, 243, 269
Vitamin D, 258
Vitamin deficiencies, 167
Vitamin E, 153
Vitamins, 167–68. See also specific type

W

Wasabi
  ulcer prevention and, 164
  Wasabi Sesame Salmon with Brown Rice Noodles, 143, 253
Water intake, 107, 108, 120
Water loss, 107

Watermelon
  Blue Ribbon Cheese Burger, 144
  California Fruit Kebabs, 269
  Cheese and Veggie Quesadilla, 142
  Veggie Delight Scramble, 132
Weight gain, 73
Weight loss. See also Skinny Chicks programme
  alcohol and, 112
  blood sugar levels and, 9, 12
  calcium and, 73
  dietary fat and, 92–94
  essential fatty acids and, 98
  negative thinking and, 55
  PC Combo and, 68
  pitfalls of, 30–31, 34
  protein and, 68–69
  protein/carb/fats formula and, 85
  questions about in Skinny Chicks programme, 56
  salads and, 7–9
  semi-starvation theory of, 27–28, 30
  Skinny Chicks programme and, 117, 207
  starvation theory of, 18, 24–27
  successful, 7
  supplements for, 173–74
Workouts
  advanced, 190–95, 197, 197–99, 200, 200
  beginner, 181–86, 181, 185–86
  guidelines, 196
  intermediate, 186–87, 187–89, 189

Y

Yogurt
  Apple Maple Pecan Parfait, 138
  Blueberry Yogurt Parfait with Slivered Almonds, 150
  California Fruit Kebabs, 135, 269
  Christine's High-Protein Pumpkin Ginger Pancakes, 237
  Citrus-y Greek Yogurt, 127, 145
  Fruity Bagel Dippers, 153
  Greek Yogurt with Honey and Walnuts, 163
  Hard-Boiled Eggs, Yogurt and Fruit, 125
  Honey Nut Apple Crunch, 158
  Pomegranate Blueberry Greek Yogurt, 122
  Raspberry Chambord Trifle, 273
  Steel-Cut (Scotch) Oats with Side of Sweet Yogurt, 34
  types, comparison of, 70, 71
  Wild Berry Parfait, 126
'You are what you think' concept, 55, 60